PANCREATITIS
DIET COOKBOOK

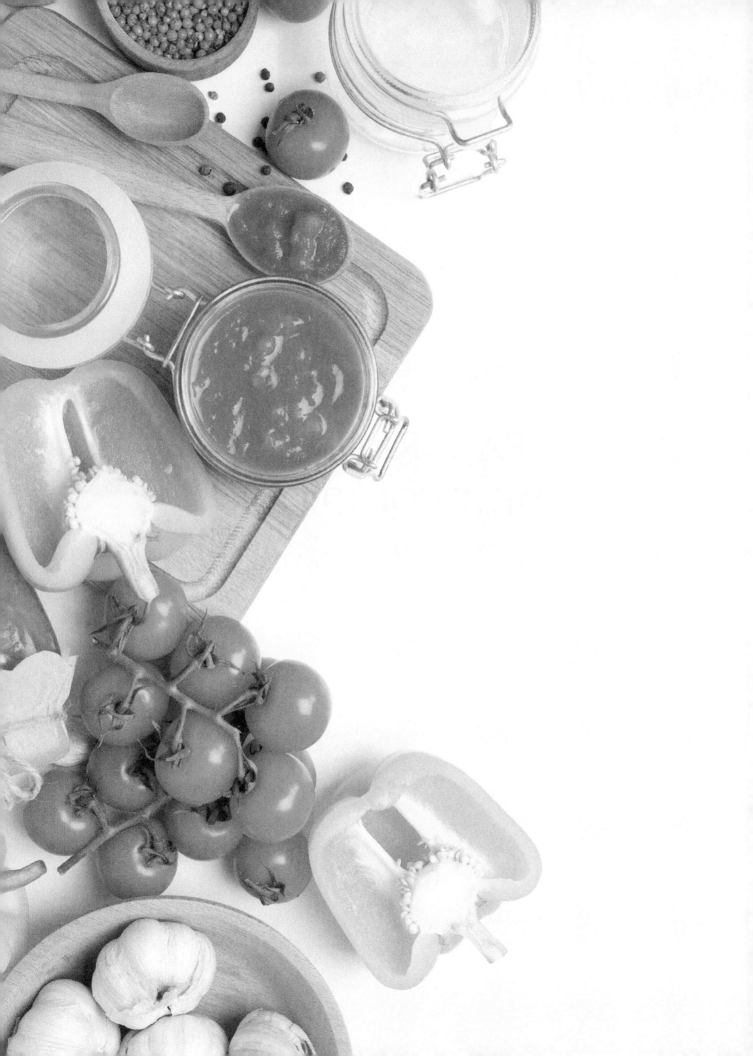

PANCREATITIS DIET COOKBOOK

1800 Days of Nutrient-Rich, Healthy, Tasty Recipes for Control Chronic Pancreatitis & Reduce Inflammation and Pain. Includes a 28-Day Meal Plan

AMANDA RAY

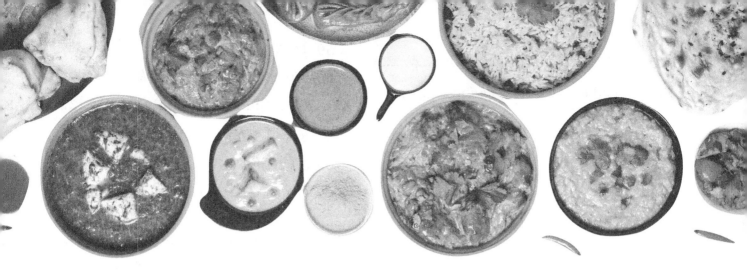

TABLE OF CONTENT

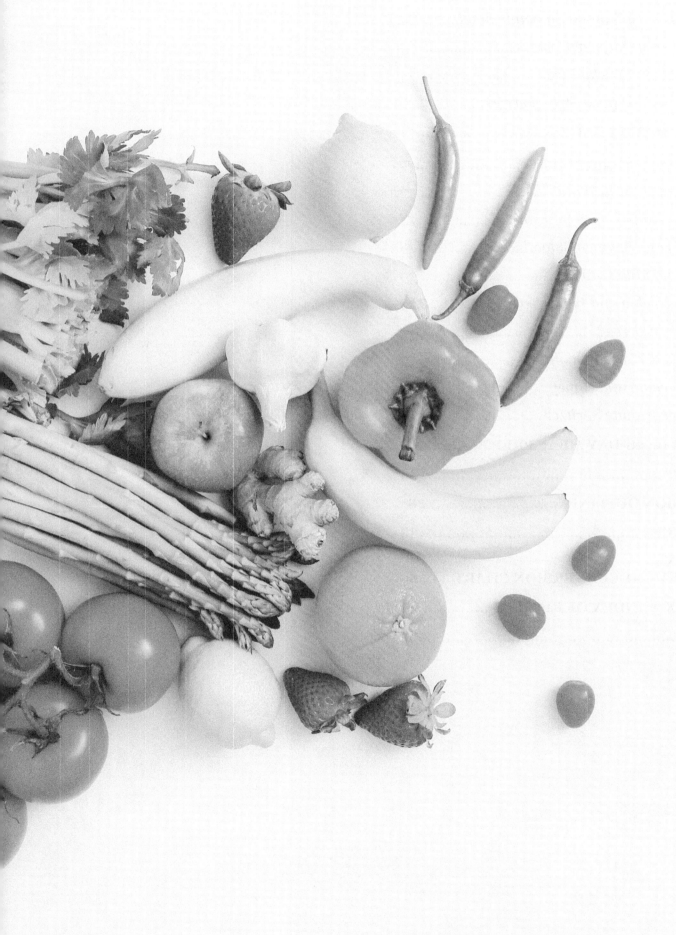

INTRODUCTION

Welcome to a fresh start on your journey with pancreatitis. As a professional nutritionist and cook, I understand that navigating the dietary needs for pancreatitis can be challenging. This Pancreatitis Diet Cookbook for Beginners is designed to simplify that journey, offering you a guide to meals that are not only safe and nutritious but also delicious.

Living with pancreatitis requires carefully balancing the proper nutrients to support your pancreas, while avoiding those that can cause irritation or exacerbate symptoms. This cookbook aims to provide you with an array of recipes that respect these principles, focusing on low-fat, high-protein foods and cooking methods that preserve the integrity of the ingredients while minimizing the use of fats.

From the basics of understanding your condition and its dietary implications to mastering the art of preparing pancreas-friendly meals, this cookbook is your companion. It will help you prevent malnutrition, manage your blood sugar levels, and potentially avoid further episodes of pancreatitis.

Each recipe has been carefully crafted with your health in mind, avoiding high-fat ingredients like fried foods and butter and incorporating beneficial spices like turmeric and ginger. Whether you're in the mood for a comforting soup or a hearty main dish, you'll find options here that satisfy your cravings without compromising your health.

Embrace this new way of cooking and eating as a positive step towards managing your pancreatitis. Let's make every meal a building block towards better health and well-being.

Greetings! My name is Amanda Ray, and I am a seasoned cookbook author with extensive expertise in the culinary world. I wanted to thank you for grabbing a copy of my diet cookbook. Your support means the world to me.

Creating this cookbook was an actual passion project for me. I wanted to make something that tastes amazing and helps people care for their health better. It's all about making those small steps towards a healthier lifestyle, and having you on board makes it all worthwhile.

I've put a lot of heart and soul into crafting these recipes, knowing how important it is to make healthy eating delicious and accessible. With so many health issues cropping up at younger ages, paying attention to what we eat is more crucial than ever.

Your decision to try out the recipes in this cookbook is a vote of confidence in my mission, and I'm genuinely grateful for that. I hope you enjoy cooking and eating from it as much as I enjoyed putting it together.

If you have a spare moment, I'd love to hear your thoughts on the cookbook. Your feedback could be super helpful for others thinking about giving it a try. Just a few words from you could make a big difference in someone else's decision-making process.

Just 3 easy steps to share your thoughts:

1. Head over to Your Orders.

2. Click "Write a product review" in the Customer Reviews section.

3. Choose a rating, and feel free to add any text, photos, or videos you'd like. Then, hit Submit!

Once again, thank you so much for your support and trust. I hope this cookbook brings you extra joy and health.

CHAPTER 1: MASTERING PANCREATITIS MANAGEMENT

Welcome to Chapter 1 of your journey into the world of pancreatitis management through diet. As a nutritionist and cook, I'm here to guide you through the basics of eating well to support your pancreas.

Understanding Your Pancreas

Your pancreas is a vital organ that aids in digestion and regulates blood sugar. When it becomes inflamed, which happens in pancreatitis, it's crucial to adjust your diet to ease its workload.

The Role of Diet in Pancreatitis

The food you eat plays a significant role in managing pancreatitis. A well-crafted diet can help prevent flare-ups, provide the nutrients needed for healing, and manage or prevent complications like diabetes.

What to Eat

Focus on high-protein, nutrient-dense foods. Lean proteins such as chicken, turkey, and fish are excellent choices. Incorporate a variety of fruits and vegetables for vitamins and minerals. Whole grains provide fiber, which can aid digestion.

What to Avoid

Foods high in fat, incredibly saturated fats, can trigger pancreatitis symptoms. This means steering clear of fried foods, full-fat dairy, and fatty cuts of meat. Also, avoid alcohol, as it can be particularly harmful to your pancreas.

Cooking for Your Pancreas

Cooking methods matter. Baking, grilling, steaming, and boiling are preferable to frying. Use herbs and spices for flavor instead of butter or oil.

Supplementing with Enzymes

Your doctor may prescribe pancreatic enzymes to help with digestion. Take them as directed to get the most benefit from the food you eat.

The Importance of Hydration

Staying hydrated is essential. Water helps with digestion and nutrient absorption, so aim for at least eight glasses a day.

Monitoring Blood Sugar

If you have pancreatitis, you're at a higher risk for diabetes. Monitor your blood sugar levels and choose complex carbohydrates over simple sugars.

In summary, managing pancreatitis with diet involves eating the right foods correctly. Stick to lean proteins, fruits, vegetables, and whole grains. Avoid high-fat foods and alcohol, and stay hydrated. Remember, this is a positive step towards better health.

1.1. UNDERSTANDING PANCREATITIS

Role and Function of the Pancreas

Welcome to the first step in understanding how your pancreas affects your health and how your diet can support this vital organ. The pancreas may be small, but it plays a huge role in your body's overall function, especially in digestion and blood sugar regulation.

The Pancreas: A Dual-Function Organ

Your pancreas is a multitasker. It has two main jobs: helping in digestion (exocrine function) and controlling blood sugar (endocrine function). For digestion, it makes enzymes that break down the foods you eat so your body can absorb the nutrients it needs. For blood sugar regulation, it produces insulin, which helps your body use or store the glucose you get from food.

When Pancreatitis Strikes

Pancreatitis is when the pancreas becomes inflamed. This can happen suddenly or over many years. In both cases, it's often painful and can lead to serious health issues. It's important to understand that during pancreatitis, your pancreas can't do its jobs as well as it should.

Diet's Role in Pancreatitis

With pancreatitis, what you eat becomes even more critical. You need to choose foods that won't overwork your pancreas. This means foods that are easy to digest and don't cause spikes in blood sugar.

The Power of Nutrition

A well-planned diet can help your pancreas heal and prevent further damage. It can also reduce your risk of developing diabetes, which can be a complication of chronic pancreatitis. By focusing on the right foods and avoiding the wrong ones, you're taking a big step in managing your condition.

In this chapter, we'll dive deeper into the pancreas's functions and how pancreatitis can change them. You'll learn how to support your pancreas through diet and lifestyle changes that can make a real difference in your health.

Remember, you're not alone on this journey. With knowledge and the right tools, you can take control of your pancreatitis and lead a healthier, happier life.

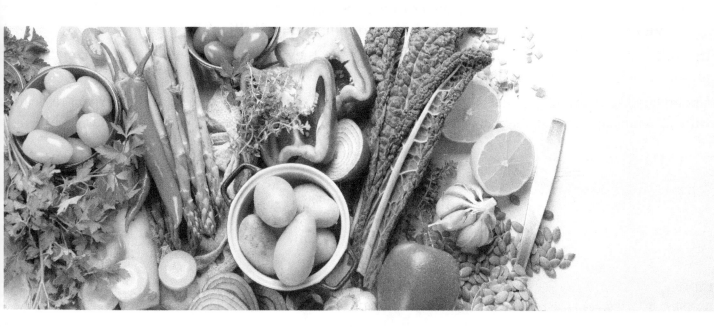

Differences Between Acute and Chronic Pancreatitis

Initially, we'll explore the differences between acute and chronic pancreatitis, which are important to know as they influence your diet and management of the condition.

Acute Pancreatitis: The Sudden Onset

Acute pancreatitis is like a sudden storm. It appears quickly, often triggered by gallstones or heavy alcohol use, and causes severe pain in the upper abdomen. It's a one-time event for some, but for others it may recur and eventually lead to chronic pancreatitis.

Eating might be the last thing on your mind during an acute attack, as treatment often involves fasting to rest the pancreas. When you start eating again, choosing foods that are gentle on your digestive system is crucial.

Chronic Pancreatitis: The Long Haul

Chronic pancreatitis, on the other hand, is a long-lasting inflammation of the pancreas. It develops over the years and can result from repeated episodes of acute pancreatitis or ongoing damage from alcohol and other causes. Unlike the acute form, chronic pancreatitis can lead to permanent damage and affects not only your digestion but also your ability to produce insulin.

With chronic pancreatitis, your diet is your daily tool for managing symptoms and preventing malnutrition. It's all about consistent, pancreas-friendly eating habits that support your body's needs without overburdening your pancreas.

The Dietary Divide

For both types of pancreatitis, alcohol is a no-go. It's harmful to your pancreas and can trigger attacks. But there are some differences in dietary approaches:

Acute Pancreatitis:

- Short-term fasting may be necessary.
- Gradually reintroduce a low-fat, high-protein diet.
- Stay hydrated with clear liquids.

Chronic Pancreatitis:

- Consistent, low-fat meals are crucial.
- You may need enzyme supplements to aid digestion.
- Vitamins and minerals might be necessary to combat malnutrition.

In both cases, avoiding high-fat foods is essential, as they can strain your pancreas. Opt for lean proteins, fruits, vegetables, and whole grains instead.

Understanding these differences helps you adapt your diet to your body's needs. Whether you're dealing with an acute episode or managing chronic pancreatitis, what you eat plays a vital role in your well-being.

Causes and Symptoms

Embarking on a journey to manage pancreatitis through diet also initiates with understanding the causes and recognizing the symptoms of this condition. This chapter aims to demystify pancreatitis, offering a foundation for why dietary choices are crucial in managing your health.

What Causes Pancreatitis?

Pancreatitis occurs when the pancreas becomes inflamed. Several factors can contribute to this inflammation:

1. **Gallstones:** These are the leading cause of acute pancreatitis. They can block the duct through which pancreatic enzymes exit, causing these enzymes to attack the pancreas itself.
2. **Alcohol:** Heavy alcohol consumption is a common cause of both acute and chronic pancreatitis.
3. **Medications:** Certain drugs can induce pancreatitis as a side effect.
4. **High Triglyceride Levels:** Elevated levels of these fats in the blood can lead to pancreatitis.
5. **Abdominal Injury:** Trauma to the abdomen may cause pancreatitis.
6. **Infections:** Various infections can precipitate an inflamed pancreas.
7. **Genetic Disorders:** In some cases, genetic factors can make an individual more susceptible to pancreatitis.

Recognizing the Symptoms

The symptoms of pancreatitis can vary depending on whether the condition is acute or chronic.

Acute Pancreatitis Symptoms:

- Sudden, severe pain in the upper abdomen
- Pain that radiates to the back
- Pain that worsens after eating
- Nausea and vomiting
- Fever and an increased heart rate

Chronic Pancreatitis Symptoms:

- Upper abdominal pain
- Weight loss without trying
- Oily, smelly stools (steatorrhea)
- Diabetes symptoms, such as increased thirst and urination

It's important to note that chronic pancreatitis symptoms may not be as noticeable at first but can become more persistent as the condition progresses.

Diet's Impact on Pancreatitis

Understanding the causes and symptoms of pancreatitis underscores the importance of diet in managing this condition. By avoiding certain triggers and focusing on nutrient-rich foods, you can help to reduce the burden on your pancreas and alleviate symptoms.

In the following chapters, we will delve into the specifics of a pancreatitis-friendly diet, offering recipes and tips to nourish your body and support your pancreas.

1.2. NUTRITIONAL MANAGEMENT

Foods to Embrace for Pancreatic Health

Navigating your diet after a pancreatitis diagnosis can feel overwhelming, but it doesn't have to be. This chapter is your guide to embracing foods that support pancreatic health and contribute to your overall well-being.

The Pancreas-Friendly Plate

When you have pancreatitis, your pancreas needs tender loving care, and your food is critical. A pancreas-friendly plate is rich in nutrients, low in fat, and includes a variety of foods that are easy to digest.

Here's what to focus on:

1. **Fruits and Vegetables:** Nature's Bounty Fruits and vegetables are packed with vitamins, minerals, and antioxidants that can help reduce inflammation. Go for a rainbow of colors to maximize the variety of nutrients. Steaming or baking vegetables makes them easier to digest.

2. **Lean Proteins:** Building Blocks for Healing Protein is essential for repairing and building tissues. Choose lean options like chicken, turkey, and fish. Plant-based proteins such as beans and lentils are also excellent choices and are less taxing on the pancreas.

3. **Whole Grains:** Sustained Energy Whole grains provide fiber, which can help regulate your digestive system without overworking your pancreas. Options like brown rice, quinoa, and whole-grain bread are great staples for your pantry.

4. **Low-Fat Dairy Alternatives:** Gentle on the Gut Dairy can be complex on a sensitive pancreas, so opt for low-fat or fat-free options. Better yet, try plant-based alternatives like almond milk or coconut yogurt, which are typically easier to digest.

5. **Healthy Fats:** Essential in Moderation While you should limit fats, your body still needs them. Focus on healthy sources like avocados, nuts, and seeds. Remember, moderation is key—too much fat can aggravate your pancreas.

Hydration: The Foundation of Health

Water is crucial for all aspects of health, including pancreatic function. Stay well-hydrated throughout the day to help your pancreas and the rest of your body work smoothly.

Creating Your Pancreatitis-Friendly Kitchen

Stock your kitchen with these pancreas-friendly foods, and you'll always have the ingredients for a healthy meal. Planning ahead and preparing meals that align with these guidelines can help you manage your symptoms and nourish your body.

Remember, each person's needs can vary, so it's essential to work with a healthcare provider or dietitian to create a diet plan that's tailored to you.

As you embrace these foods, you'll not only support your pancreas but also embark on a path to a healthier lifestyle. Bon appétit!

Foods to Avoid to Prevent Flare-ups

When you're navigating life with pancreatitis, knowing which foods to avoid is just as important as knowing which foods to embrace. Steering clear of certain foods can help prevent painful flare-ups and manage your condition effectively.

High-Fat Foods: The Heavy Hitters

Fatty foods are tough on the pancreas, requiring more work to digest. This can exacerbate pancreatitis and lead to discomfort. Here's what to skip:

1. **Fried and Greasy Foods:** Avoid fried chicken, french fries, and other greasy delights.
2. **Full-Fat Dairy:** Whole milk, cream, and cheese can be too rich for your sensitive pancreas.
3. **Fatty Meats:** Avoid cuts of meat with visible fat and skin, such as pork belly or duck.

Alcohol: The Inflammatory Ingredient

Alcohol can cause significant inflammation in the pancreas and is a common trigger for acute pancreatitis. It's best to eliminate alcohol entirely to protect your pancreatic health.

Refined Carbohydrates: The Sugar Spike

Foods high in refined sugars and flour can cause blood sugar levels to spike, which is something you want to avoid, especially if you have pancreatitis. Limit or avoid:

1. **Sugary Snacks:** Candies, cookies, and cakes are off the menu.
2. **White Bread and Pasta:** Opt for their whole-grain counterparts instead.

Spicy Foods: The Hidden Agitators

While not universally problematic, spicy foods can irritate some people's pancreatitis. If you find that spicy meals trigger your symptoms, it's wise to avoid them.

Caffeine: The Controversial Stimulant

Caffeine's impact on pancreatitis isn't clear-cut, but it can affect digestion and may exacerbate symptoms for some. Monitor how your body reacts to caffeine and consider cutting back if necessary.

Putting It All Together

Creating a diet plan that avoids these foods can significantly reduce the risk of pancreatitis flare-ups. Remember, moderation is essential, and occasional indulgences should be carefully considered in consultation with your healthcare provider.

Importance of Hydration

In the landscape of managing pancreatitis, hydration stands as a cornerstone. This chapter highlights the critical role of water in the diet of individuals with pancreatitis and offers practical advice for maintaining optimal hydration.

Why Hydration Matters

Water is the lifeblood of our cells, the transporter of nutrients, and the medium through which our body's processes occur. For those with pancreatitis, staying hydrated is especially important because it helps:

1. **Maintain Pancreatic Function:** Adequate hydration supports the pancreas in producing digestive enzymes and hormones effectively.
2. **Ease Digestion:** Water helps break down food, allowing for easier digestion and less strain on the pancreas.
3. **Reduce Inflammation:** Proper hydration can help to reduce inflammation throughout the body, including the pancreas.
4. **Flush Toxins:** Adequate water intake helps the kidneys remove waste products, vital as the pancreas heals.

How Much Water Should You Drink?

The amount of water each person needs can vary based on factors like age, weight, climate, and activity level. However, a general guideline for adults is to aim for 8-10 glasses (64–80 ounces) of water daily. It's important to listen to your body and drink more if you're feeling thirsty or if your urine is dark, which can indicate dehydration.

Tips for Staying Hydrated

1. Start your day with a glass of water to kick-start hydration.
2. Keep a reusable water bottle with you throughout the day to make it easier to drink water regularly.
3. If you find plain water unappealing, add a slice of lemon or lime for flavor.
4. Eat water-rich foods like cucumbers, watermelon, and oranges, contributing to your daily fluid intake.
5. Set reminders on your phone or use a hydration-tracking app to ensure you drink enough water.

Remember, while water is the best choice for hydration, other fluids like herbal teas can also contribute to your daily intake. However, beverages containing caffeine or alcohol should be avoided or limited, as they can lead to dehydration.

Hydration is a simple yet powerful tool in your pancreatitis management toolkit. By ensuring you adequately hydrated, you're taking an essential step in supporting your pancreas and your overall health.

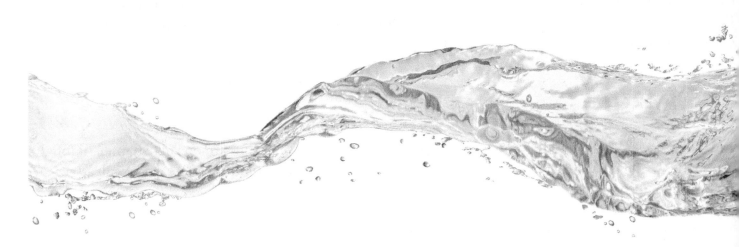

1.3. LIFESTYLE ADJUSTMENTS

Benefits and Recommendations for Physical Activity

In addition to dietary changes, physical activity is essential for treating pancreatitis and enhancing general health and wellbeing. This chapter will examine the advantages of physical activity for people with pancreatitis and offer helpful suggestions for integrating physical activity into your daily routine safely.

The Advantages of Exercise

For various reasons, exercise is vital in the treatment of pancreatitis.

1. **Weight management:** Keeping your weight within a healthy range eases the burden on your pancreas and digestive system.
2. **Better Digestion:** Regular physical activity can help lessen pancreatitis symptoms and support a healthy digestive system.
3. **Enhanced Mood:** Exercise releases endorphins, which have the power to elevate mood and lower stress levels. Stress is a major factor because it can aggravate the symptoms of pancreatitis.
4. **Enhanced Insulin Sensitivity:** Exercise can help control blood sugar levels and to improve insulin sensitivity in people who are at risk of diabetes as a result of chronic pancreatitis.

Guidelines for Physical Exercise

It's important to start cautiously and pick enjoyable activities when adding fitness to your regimen. The following suggestions are provided:

1. **Start with Low-Impact Exercises:** Cycling, walking, and swimming are great low-impact workouts that can cause your body to experience less stress.
2. **Gradually raise Intensity:** You can gradually increase the duration and intensity of your workouts as your fitness level rises.
3. **Pay Attention to Your Body:** Observe how your body reacts to physical activity. If you feel pain or discomfort, stop, talk to your doctor, and take a break.
4. **Remain Steady:** Health officials advise engaging in at least 150 minutes of moderate-intensity exercise every week.

Safety Measures and Advice

Exercise is good however there are certain things to be careful of:

1. **Refrain from High-Intensity Exercise During Flare-Ups:** Rest is essential when experiencing acute pancreatitis. Resuming exercise should only be done with your doctor's approval.
2. **Keep Yourself Hydrated:** To avoid being dehydrated during or after exercise, sip lots of water.
3. **Fuel Your Body:** Follow the advice in your customized pancreatitis diet plan to have a balanced meal or snack to make sure you have adequate energy for your activities.

To sum up, maintaining a regular physical activity regimen is crucial for treating pancreatitis. You may take care of your pancreatic health and reap the advantages of exercise at the same time by adhering to these suggestions and consulting with your healthcare provider.

Strategies for Managing Cravings and Making Healthy Substitutes

When you're adapting to a pancreatitis-friendly diet, cravings for off-limits foods can be one of the biggest hurdles. But fear not! With a few innovative strategies and creative substitutes, you can satisfy those cravings without compromising your health. Here's how to navigate your desires and maintain a pancreatitis-safe diet.

Understanding Cravings

Firstly, it's essential to understand why we crave certain foods. Cravings can be emotional, stemming from stress or habit, or they can be physiological, signaling nutritional deficiencies or fluctuations in blood sugar levels. Recognizing the root cause of your cravings can help you address them effectively.

Healthy Substitutes for Common Cravings

1. **For a creamy texture:** Instead of high-fat dairy products, opt for fat-free Greek yogurt or mashed avocado. These provide a creamy consistency while being kinder to your pancreas.
2. **Sweet treats:** Craving something sweet? Reach for fresh fruit like berries or a small serving of dried fruit. These natural sugars are pancreas-friendly when enjoyed in moderation.
3. **Salty snacks:** Rather than grabbing chips, try air-popped popcorn seasoned with a sprinkle of nutritional yeast or herbs for that satisfying crunch without the added fats.
4. **Chocolate:** If chocolate is your weakness, choose dark chocolate with a high cocoa content in small amounts. It's lower in sugar and fat compared to milk chocolate.

Strategies to Manage Cravings

1. **Stay hydrated:** Sometimes, what we perceive as hunger is actually thirst. Drink a glass of water and wait a few minutes to see if the craving subsides.
2. **Distract yourself:** Engage in an enjoyable activity to take your mind off the craving. A brisk walk, a puzzle, or calling a friend can help.
3. **Plan your meals:** Having a structured meal plan can reduce impulsive eating and help you stick to pancreatitis-friendly foods.
4. **Portion control:** If you decide to indulge in a craving, do so mindfully and in small portions to avoid triggering a flare-up.

Remember, it's about balance and making informed choices. By incorporating these strategies and substitutes into your lifestyle, you can manage your cravings while supporting your pancreas and overall health.

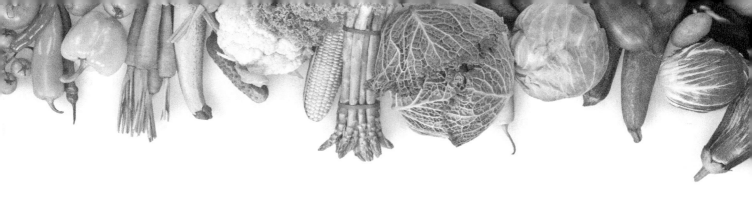

CHAPTER 2: BREAKFASTS

1. Apple-Cinnamon Oat Porridge

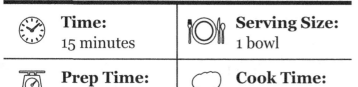

⏰ **Time:** 15 minutes	🍽 **Serving Size:** 1 bowl
⚖ **Prep Time:** 5 minutes	👨‍🍳 **Cook Time:** 10 minutes

Nutrition Information Per Serving (1 bowl):

Calories: 150, Carbohydrates: 27g, Saturated Fat: 0.5g, Protein: 4g, Fat: 2.5g, Sodium: 50mg, Potassium: 163mg, Fiber: 4g, Sugar: 10g, Vitamin C: 2mg, Calcium: 20mg, Iron: 1.2mg

Ingredients:

- 1/2 cup rolled oats
- 1 cup water or low-fat milk
- 1 medium apple, peeled and diced
- 1/4 teaspoon ground cinnamon
- 1 teaspoon honey (optional)
- Pinch of salt

Directions:

1. Bring one cup of water or low-fat milk to a boil in a small pot. Sprinkle in some salt.
2. Stir in 1/2 cup rolled oats and reduce heat to a simmer.
3. Add the diced apple and 1/4 teaspoon ground cinnamon to the saucepan.
4. Cook, stirring periodically, until the porridge thickens to your desired consistency and the oats are soft, about 10 minutes.
5. Remove from heat and let it cool slightly. If desired, stir in 1 teaspoon of honey for a touch of sweetness.
6. Serve warm and enjoy your Apple-Cinnamon Oat Porridge.

2. Quinoa Breakfast Bowl with Berries

⏰ **Time:** 25 minutes	🍽 **Serving Size:** 1 bowl
⚖ **Prep Time:** 5 minutes	👨‍🍳 **Cook Time:** 20 minutes

Nutrition Information Per Serving (1 bowl):

Calories: 285, Carbohydrates: 52g, Saturated Fat: 0.5g, Protein: 8g, Fat: 5g, Sodium: 13mg, Potassium: 320mg, Fiber: 6g, Sugar: 8g, Vitamin C: 1.2mg, Calcium: 30mg, Iron: 2.5mg

Ingredients:

- 1/2 cup quinoa, rinsed
- 1 cup water
- 1/2 cup fresh berries (strawberries, blueberries, or raspberries)
- 1 tablespoon chopped nuts (almonds or walnuts, optional)
- 1 tablespoon honey or maple syrup (optional)
- A pinch of cinnamon (optional)

Directions:

1. Pour one cup of water and half a cup of rinsed quinoa into a small pot. Heat to a boil on a medium-high heat setting.

2. Once boiling, reduce the heat to low, cover, and simmer for about 15 to 20 minutes, or until the quinoa is cooked and the water is absorbed.

3. While the quinoa is cooking, rinse 1/2 cup of fresh berries and set aside.

4. If using nuts, roughly chop 1 tablespoon of almonds or walnuts.

5. When the quinoa is done, remove from heat and let it sit covered for 5 minutes. Then fluff it with a fork.

6. Place the cooked quinoa in a bowl for serving. Place the chopped nuts and fresh berries on top, if desired.

7. If preferred, drizzle with 1 tablespoon of maple syrup or honey for a little sweetness. Sprinkle a pinch of cinnamon over the top for added flavor.

8. Serve the Quinoa Breakfast Bowl warm and enjoy a nutritious start to your day.

3. Spinach and Feta Egg Muffins

⏰ **Time:** 30 minutes	🍽 **Serving Size:** 1 plate
⚖ **Prep Time:** 10 minutes	👨‍🍳 **Cook Time:** 20 minutes

Nutrition Information Per Serving (1 plate):

Calories: 120, Carbohydrates: 3g, Saturated Fat: 2g, Protein: 9g, Fat: 7g, Sodium: 200mg, Potassium: 160mg, Fiber: 1g, Sugar: 1g, Vitamin C: 4mg, Calcium: 110mg, Iron: 1.5mg

Ingredients:

- 3 egg whites
- 1/2 cup fresh spinach, chopped
- 1/4 cup feta cheese, crumbled
- 1 tablespoon skim milk
- Salt and pepper to taste
- Cooking spray

Directions:

1. Adjust the oven temperature to 350°F. Lightly coat a muffin tray with cooking spray.

2. Whisk the egg whites, skim milk, salt, and pepper in a mixing dish.

3. Add the chopped spinach to the egg mixture and stir to combine.

4. Halfway full, pour the egg and spinach mixture into each cup of the muffin pan that has been prepared.

5. Sprinkle the crumbled feta cheese evenly over each muffin cup.

6. After 20 minutes, or when the egg muffins are set and have a light golden color on top, place the muffin tin in the oven.

7. Take out the muffin tin from the oven, then let the muffins cool for a few minutes to cool before taking them out of the pan.

8. Serve the Spinach and Feta Egg Muffins warm, and enjoy your nutritious, pancreatitis-friendly breakfast!

4. Banana and Walnut Smoothie

⏰ **Time:** 10 minutes	🍽 **Serving Size:** 1 glass
⚖ **Prep Time:** 5 minutes	👨‍🍳 **Cook Time:** 5 minutes

Nutrition Information Per Serving (1 glass):

Calories: 220, Carbohydrates: 27g, Saturated Fat: 0.6g, Protein: 6g, Fat: 11g, Sodium: 20mg, Potassium: 450mg, Fiber: 3g, Sugar: 14g, Vitamin C: 7mg, Calcium: 20mg, Iron: 0.7mg

Ingredients:

- 1/2 cup almond milk, unsweetened
- 1/4 teaspoon vanilla extract
- A pinch of ground cinnamon
- 1 ripe banana
- 2 tablespoons chopped walnuts
- 1/2 cup low-fat Greek yogurt
- Ice cubes (optional)

Directions:

1. Peel 1 ripe banana and place it into a blender.
2. Add 2 tablespoons of chopped walnuts to the blender.
3. Incorporate 1/2 cup of low-fat Greek yogurt for protein.
4. To make a creamy base, stir in 1/2 cup of unsweetened almond milk.
5. Add 1/4 teaspoon of vanilla extract for flavor.
6. Sprinkle a pinch of ground cinnamon for a touch of warmth.
7. For a cold smoothie, feel free to add a handful of ice cubes to the blender.
8. On high, blend all the ingredients until they are creamy and smooth.
9. Pour the smoothie into a glass and enjoy your nourishing breakfast.

5. Greek Yogurt with Honey and Almonds

⏰	**Time:** 5 minutes	🍽	**Serving Size:** 1 bowl
⚖	**Prep Time:** 5 minutes	👨‍🍳	**Cook Time:** 0 minutes

Nutrition Information Per Serving (1 bowl):

Calories: 150, Carbohydrates: 18g, Saturated Fat: 0g, Protein: 10g, Fat: 4g, Sodium: 50mg, Potassium: 200mg, Fiber: 1g, Sugar: 17g, Vitamin C: 0mg, Calcium: 150mg, Iron: 0.5mg

Ingredients:

- 3/4 cup low-fat Greek yogurt
- 1 tablespoon honey
- 2 tablespoons sliced almonds

Directions:

1. Place 3/4 cup of low-fat Greek yogurt into a serving bowl.
2. Drizzle 1 tablespoon of honey over the Greek yogurt.
3. Sprinkle 2 tablespoons of sliced almonds on top of the yogurt and honey.
4. Gently mix the honey and almonds with the yogurt if preferred, or leave them layered.
5. Serve immediately and enjoy this simple yet nutritious breakfast.

6. Sweet Potato and Kale Hash

🕐	**Time:** 35 minutes	🍽️	**Serving Size:** 1 plate
⚖️	**Prep Time:** 15 minutes	👨‍🍳	**Cook Time:** 20 minutes

Nutrition Information Per Serving (1 plate):

Calories: 200, Carbohydrates: 38g, Saturated Fat: 0.5g, Protein: 4g, Fat: 3g, Sodium: 70mg, Potassium: 670mg, Fiber: 6g, Sugar: 7g, Vitamin C: 19mg, Calcium: 76mg, Iron: 1.4mg

Ingredients:

- 1 medium sweet potato, peeled and diced
- 1 cup kale, washed and chopped
- 1/4 cup red onion, finely chopped
- 1/2 teaspoon olive oil
- 1/4 teaspoon garlic powder
- Salt and pepper to taste
- Fresh parsley for garnish (optional)

Directions:

1. Preheat your oven to 400°F.
2. Spread the diced sweet potato on a baking sheet and drizzle with 1/2 teaspoon of olive oil. Season with salt, pepper, and 1/4 teaspoon of garlic powder.
3. Sweet potatoes should be baked for about 20 minutes, stirring halfway through, or until they are soft.
4. Set a nonstick skillet over medium heat while the sweet potatoes roast.
5. When the red onion is diced and added to the skillet, sauté it for about three minutes, or until it turns transparent.
6. When the kale is soft and wilted, add it to the skillet with the onions and simmer for about five minutes.
7. Once the sweet potatoes are done, add them to the skillet with the onions and kale, and toss to combine.
8. Serve the hash warm, garnished with fresh parsley if desired.

7. Cottage Cheese with Pineapple Chunks

🕐	**Time:** 15 minutes	🍽️	**Serving Size:** 1 bowl
⚖️	**Prep Time:** 5 minutes	👨‍🍳	**Cook Time:** 10 minutes

Nutrition Information Per Serving (1 bowl):

Calories: 150, Carbohydrates: 15g, Saturated Fat: 1g, Protein: 14g, Fat: 2g, Sodium: 500mg, Potassium: 200mg, Fiber: 1g, Sugar: 13g, Vitamin C: 10mg, Calcium: 125mg, Iron: 0.3mg

Ingredients:

- 1/2 cup low-fat cottage cheese
- 1/2 cup pineapple chunks, fresh or canned in juice
- 1 tablespoon sliced almonds (optional)
- A pinch of cinnamon (optional)

Directions:

1. Place the low-fat cottage cheese in a serving bowl.
2. If using canned pineapple, drain the juice to remove excess sugar. Add the pineapple chunks on top of the cottage cheese.
3. For added texture and nutrients, sprinkle sliced almonds over the cottage cheese and pineapple.
4. If desired, add a pinch of cinnamon for flavor.
5. Serve immediately and enjoy this refreshing and protein-rich breakfast.

8. Pumpkin Spice Oatmeal

	Time: 20 minutes		Serving Size: 1 bowl
	Prep Time: 5 minutes		Cook Time: 15 minutes

Nutrition Information Per Serving (1 bowl):

Calories: 280, Carbohydrates: 51g, Saturated Fat: 0.5g, Protein: 10g, Fat: 4g, Sodium: 80mg, Potassium: 250mg, Fiber: 6g, Sugar: 12g, Vitamin C: 2mg, Calcium: 20mg, Iron: 2.5mg

Ingredients:

- 1/2 cup rolled oats
- 1 cup water
- 1/4 cup pumpkin puree
- 1/4 teaspoon pumpkin pie spice
- 1 tablespoon maple syrup
- 1/4 teaspoon vanilla extract
- Pinch of salt
- 2 tablespoons low-fat milk or a milk substitute

Directions:

1. Heat one cup of water in a small pot until it boils. After adding 1/2 cup of rolled oats and a pinch of salt, lower the heat to a simmer.

2. Cook the oats for about 10-15 minutes, stirring occasionally, until they have absorbed the water and reached your desired consistency.

3. Stir in 1/4 cup pumpkin puree, 1/4 teaspoon pumpkin pie spice, 1 tablespoon maple syrup, and 1/4 teaspoon vanilla extract into the cooked oatmeal.

4. Cook for another minute or two, until everything is heated and well combined.

5. Pour the oatmeal into a bowl and drizzle with 2 tablespoons of low-fat milk or your choice of milk substitute.

6. Serve hot and enjoy your Pumpkin Spice Oatmeal, a comforting and pancreatitis-friendly breakfast option!

9. Scrambled Tofu with Spinach and Tomatoes

	Time: 15 minutes		Serving Size: 1 plate
	Prep Time: 5 minutes		Cook Time: 10 minutes

Nutrition Information Per Serving (1 plate):

Calories: 180, Carbohydrates: 10g, Saturated Fat: 1g, Protein: 20g, Fat: 9g, Sodium: 200mg, Potassium: 300mg, Fiber: 4g, Sugar: 3g, Vitamin C: 15mg, Calcium: 150mg, Iron: 2.5mg

Ingredients:

- 1/2 block firm tofu, drained and crumbled
- 1 cup fresh spinach, roughly chopped
- 1/2 medium tomato, diced
- 1/4 teaspoon turmeric
- 1/2 teaspoon garlic powder
- 1 tablespoon nutritional yeast
- Salt and pepper to taste
- 1 teaspoon olive oil

Directions:

1. In a nonstick skillet, warm up one teaspoon of olive oil over medium heat.

2. Add the crumbled tofu to the skillet and cook for 3-4 minutes, stirring occasionally.

3. Mix in 1/4 teaspoon turmeric and 1/2 teaspoon garlic powder to give the tofu a nice color and flavor.

4. Stir in 1 tablespoon of nutritional yeast for a cheesy taste and added nutrients.

5. Add the 1 cup of fresh spinach and cook until it begins to wilt, about 2 minutes.

6. Toss in the 1/2 diced medium tomato and cook for another 2 minutes, until the tomatoes are warmed.

7. After adding salt and pepper to taste, serve the food hot.

10. Pear and Ginger Overnight Oats

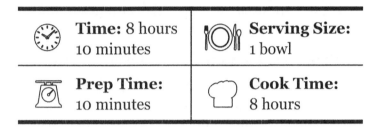

	Time: 8 hours 10 minutes		Serving Size: 1 bowl
	Prep Time: 10 minutes		Cook Time: 8 hours

Nutrition Information Per Serving (1 bowl):

Calories: 215, Carbohydrates: 38g, Saturated Fat: 0.5g, Protein: 6g, Fat: 3.5g, Sodium: 50mg, Potassium: 205mg, Fiber: 5g, Sugar: 15g, Vitamin C: 4mg, Calcium: 20mg, Iron: 1.8mg

Ingredients:

- 1/2 cup rolled oats
- 3/4 cup almond milk, unsweetened
- 1/2 pear, diced
- 1/4 teaspoon ground ginger
- 1 teaspoon honey (optional)
- 1 tablespoon chia seeds

Directions:

1. In a mason jar or a bowl, combine the rolled oats and unsweetened almond milk.

2. Stir in the chia seeds and ground ginger until well-mixed.

3. Add the diced pear to the mixture and drizzle with honey if a sweeter taste is desired.

4. Seal the jar with a lid or cover the bowl with a lid or plastic wrap.

5. Place in the refrigerator and let it sit overnight, or for at least 8 hours.

6. Stir the oats well in the morning. To get the right consistency, thin out any excess mixture by adding a small amount of almond milk.

7. Serve cold or let it sit at room temperature for a few minutes if you prefer it slightly warmer. Enjoy your nutrient-packed, pancreatitis-friendly breakfast!

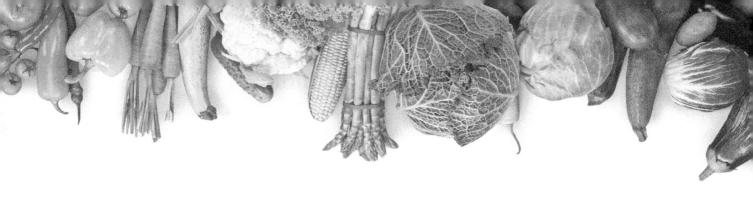

CHAPTER 3: SNACKS AND APPETIZERS

11. Carrot and Zucchini Sticks with Baba Ganoush

🕐 **Time:** 50 minutes	🍽 **Serving Size:** 1
⚖ **Prep Time:** 15 minutes	👨‍🍳 **Cook Time:** 35 minutes

Nutrition Information Per Serving (1 serving unit):

Calories: 150, Carbohydrates: 18g, Saturated Fat: 1g, Protein: 4g, Fat: 8g, Sodium: 300mg, Potassium: 450mg, Fiber: 6g, Sugar: 9g, Vitamin C: 20mg, Calcium: 50mg, Iron: 1mg

Ingredients:

- 2 medium carrots, peeled and cut into sticks
- 1 medium zucchini, cut into sticks
- 1 medium eggplant
- 2 cloves garlic, minced
- 1 tablespoon tahini
- 1 tablespoon lemon juice
- 1/4 teaspoon ground cumin
- Salt to taste
- 1 tablespoon olive oil

Directions:

1. Preheat your oven to 400°F.
2. Begin by preparing the vegetables: peel and cut the carrots into sticks, and do the same with the zucchini. Set them aside.
3. Pierce the eggplant with a fork several times and place it on a baking sheet. Bake the eggplant for 35 minutes, or until it is tender and its skin has become wrinkly.
4. Once the eggplant is roasted, allow it to cool for a few minutes, then peel off the skin and place the flesh in a food processor.
5. Add the minced garlic, tahini, lemon juice, ground cumin, and salt to the food processor with the eggplant.
6. Process until smooth, then while the processor is running, slowly drizzle in the olive oil until the mixture reaches a creamy consistency.
7. Place the baba ganoush in a dish for serving.
8. Arrange the carrot and zucchini sticks on a plate and serve with the baba ganoush for dipping.
9. Enjoy this healthy and delicious snack that's perfect for managing pancreatitis!

12. Baked Sweet Potato Fries

🕐 **Time:** 45 minutes	🍽 **Serving Size:** 2
⚖ **Prep Time:** 15 minutes	👨‍🍳 **Cook Time:** 30 minutes

Nutrition Information Per Serving (1 serving unit):

Calories: 150, Carbohydrates: 34g, Saturated Fat: 0.1g, Protein: 2g, Fat: 0.2g, Sodium: 70mg, Potassium: 474mg, Fiber: 5g, Sugar: 7g, Vitamin C: 3mg, Calcium: 43mg, Iron: 0.8mg

Ingredients:

- 2 large sweet potatoes
- 1/2 teaspoon paprika
- 1/2 teaspoon garlic powder
- 1/4 teaspoon black pepper
- 1/8 teaspoon cayenne pepper (optional)
- Cooking spray (olive oil based)

Directions:

1. Preheat your oven to 425°F.
2. To achieve equal cooking, wash and peel the sweet potatoes before cutting them into sticks that are about 1/4 inch thick.
3. In a large bowl, toss the sweet potato sticks with paprika, garlic powder, black pepper, and cayenne pepper if using, to coat evenly.
4. Apply a thin layer of cooking spray and line a baking sheet with parchment paper.
5. Arrange the sweet potato sticks in a single layer on the baking sheet, making sure they do not touch to ensure they crisp up.
6. Bake in the preheated oven for 15 minutes, then flip the fries and continue baking for another 15 minutes or until they are golden brown and crispy.
7. Take out of the oven and allow it to cool down a little before serving. Savor this tasty, pancreatitis-friendly snack!

13. Cucumber Rounds with Hummus

🕐	**Time:** 15 minutes	🍽	**Serving Size:** 4
⚖	**Prep Time:** 15 minutes	👨‍🍳	**Cook Time:** 0 minutes

Nutrition Information Per Serving (1 serving unit):

Calories: 90, Carbohydrates: 12g, Saturated Fat: 0.3g, Protein: 3g, Fat: 4.5g, Sodium: 120mg, Potassium: 230mg, Fiber: 2g, Sugar: 2g, Vitamin C: 4mg, Calcium: 30mg, Iron: 1mg

Ingredients:

- 2 large cucumbers
- 1 cup hummus
- 1 tablespoon olive oil
- 1 teaspoon paprika
- 1 tablespoon chopped parsley
- 1 clove garlic, minced
- Salt to taste

Directions:

1. Begin by washing the cucumbers thoroughly. Slice them into 1/4 inch thick rounds and set aside.
2. In a mixing bowl, combine the hummus with olive oil, minced garlic, and a pinch of salt. Mix until well incorporated.
3. Arrange the rounds of cucumber on a plate for serving.
4. Spoon a dollop of the hummus mixture onto each cucumber round.
5. Sprinkle the paprika and chopped parsley over the hummus-topped cucumber rounds for garnish.
6. Serve immediately as a fresh and healthy appetizer that's perfect for those with pancreatitis, or cover and refrigerate to keep cool until serving.

14. Fruit Salad with Mint and Lime Dressing

⏰	**Time:** 20 minutes	🍽	**Serving Size:** 4 bowls
⚖	**Prep Time:** 20 minutes	👨‍🍳	**Cook Time:** 0 minutes

Nutrition Information Per Serving (1 serving bowl):

Calories: 120, Carbohydrates: 30g, Saturated Fat: 0g, Protein: 2g, Fat: 0.5g, Sodium: 5mg, Potassium: 325mg, Fiber: 4g, Sugar: 22g, Vitamin C: 48mg, Calcium: 30mg, Iron: 0.6mg

Ingredients:

- 1 cup strawberries, hulled and sliced
- 1 cup blueberries
- 1 cup blackberries
- 1 cup green grapes, halved
- 1 large mango, peeled and diced
- 1/4 cup fresh mint leaves, finely chopped
- Juice of 2 limes
- 1 tablespoon honey (optional)
- 1 teaspoon lime zest

Directions:

1. In a large mixing bowl, combine the strawberries, blueberries, blackberries, grapes, and diced mango.

2. In a small bowl, whisk together the lime juice, honey (if using), and lime zest until well combined.

3. Drizzle the lime dressing over the mixed fruit and toss gently to coat all the fruit with the dressing.

4. Sprinkle the chopped mint over the fruit salad and toss again lightly.

5. Serve the fruit salad immediately or chill in the refrigerator for 15-30 minutes to allow the flavors to meld.

6. Enjoy this refreshing and pancreatitis-friendly snack that is both nourishing and satisfying!

15. Melon and Prosciutto Bites

⏰	**Time:** 15 minutes	🍽	**Serving Size:** 4 skewers
⚖	**Prep Time:** 15 minutes	👨‍🍳	**Cook Time:** 0 minutes

Nutrition Information Per Serving (1 skewer):

Calories: 80, Carbohydrates: 8g, Saturated Fat: 1g, Protein: 6g, Fat: 3g, Sodium: 670mg, Potassium: 194mg, Fiber: 1g, Sugar: 7g, Vitamin C: 36mg, Calcium: 11mg, Iron: 0.3mg

Ingredients:

- 1/4 cantaloupe, cut into 1-inch cubes
- 4 slices of prosciutto, cut into strips
- 1 tablespoon balsamic glaze
- Fresh basil leaves for garnish

Directions:

1. Wrap each cantaloupe cube with a strip of prosciutto.

2. Arrange the melon and prosciutto bites on a serving platter.

3. Drizzle with balsamic glaze.

4. Just before serving, add some fresh basil leaves as a garnish.

5. Enjoy as a refreshing and protein-rich appetizer.

16. Rice Paper Rolls with Avocado and Mango

⏰ **Time:** 30 minutes	🍽 **Serving Size:** 4 rolls
⚖ **Prep Time:** 20 minutes	👨‍🍳 **Cook Time:** 10 minutes

Nutrition Information Per Serving (1 roll):

Calories: 150, Carbohydrates: 28g, Saturated Fat: 1g, Protein: 4g, Fat: 4g, Sodium: 200mg, Potassium: 300mg, Fiber: 5g, Sugar: 6g, Vitamin C: 15mg, Calcium: 20mg, Iron: 1.5mg

Ingredients:

- 8 rice paper wrappers
- 1 ripe mango, peeled and cut into thin strips
- 1 avocado, peeled, pitted, and cut into thin strips
- 1 medium carrot, julienned
- 1 cucumber, julienned
- 1 cup fresh spinach
- 1/4 cup fresh cilantro leaves
- 1 tablespoon low-sodium soy sauce
- 1 tablespoon rice vinegar
- 1 teaspoon honey
- 1 teaspoon sesame oil
- Optional: 1 tablespoon crushed peanuts for garnish

Directions:

1. Tip in a big dish of warm water. One rice paper wrapper should be dipped into the water for fifteen seconds or so to make it malleable. Spread out the wrapper evenly on a fresh, moist kitchen towel.

2. In the center of the wrapper, place a small handful of spinach leaves, a few strips of mango, avocado, carrot, cucumber, and a sprinkle of cilantro leaves.

3. Once the filling is firmly covered, tuck in the sides of the wrap and keep rolling until the seam is shut.

4. Mix the soy sauce, rice vinegar, honey, and sesame oil in a small bowl to create a dipping sauce.

5. Cut the rolls in half and arrange on a serving platter. If desired, garnish with crushed peanuts.

6. Serve with the dipping sauce on the side for a refreshing and healthy snack.

17. Sliced Apples with Almond Butter

⏰ **Time:** 10 minutes	🍽 **Serving Size:** 2 apples
⚖ **Prep Time:** 10 minutes	👨‍🍳 **Cook Time:** 0 minutes

Nutrition Information Per Serving (1 apple):

Calories: 190, Carbohydrates: 25g, Saturated Fat: 0.5g, Protein: 4g, Fat: 10g, Sodium: 0mg, Potassium: 300mg, Fiber: 5g, Sugar: 17g, Vitamin C: 8mg, Calcium: 60mg, Iron: 0.5mg

Ingredients:

- 2 medium apples, any sweet variety
- 2 tablespoons almond butter, no added sugar

Directions:

1. Wash the apples thoroughly and pat them dry with a clean kitchen towel.

2. Core the apples and slice them into rounds or wedges, according to your preference.

3. Measure out the almond butter into a small dish for easy dipping.

4. Arrange the apple slices on a plate with the dish of almond butter.

5. Serve as a simple, refreshing snack or appetizer, encouraging dipping the apple slices into the almond butter for a creamy, satisfying treat.

18. Tomato Bruschetta on Whole Grain Bread

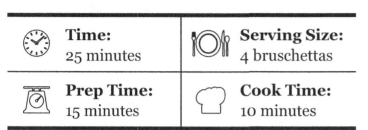 Time: 25 minutes	Serving Size: 4 bruschettas
Prep Time: 15 minutes	Cook Time: 10 minutes

Nutrition Information Per Serving (1 bruschetta):

Calories: 120, Carbohydrates: 18g, Saturated Fat: 0.2g, Protein: 4g, Fat: 3g, Sodium: 210mg, Potassium: 210mg, Fiber: 3g, Sugar: 3g, Vitamin C: 10mg, Calcium: 35mg, Iron: 1mg

Ingredients:

- 4 slices whole grain bread
- 2 medium tomatoes, finely chopped
- 1 clove garlic, minced
- 1 teaspoon olive oil
- 1 tablespoon balsamic vinegar
- 1/4 cup fresh basil leaves, chopped
- Salt and pepper to taste

Directions:

1. Preheat your oven to 350°F.
2. In a mixing bowl, combine the finely chopped tomatoes, minced garlic, olive oil, balsamic vinegar, and chopped basil. Season with salt and pepper to taste.
3. Place the whole grain bread slices on a baking sheet and toast in the oven for about 10 minutes, or until the edges are slightly crispy.
4. After taking the bread out of the oven, evenly spoon each piece with the tomato mixture.
5. Serve the bruschetta immediately while the bread is still warm and enjoy this light and flavorful appetizer.

19. Veggie Nori Rolls

Time: 25 minutes	Serving Size: 2 rolls
Prep Time: 15 minutes	Cook Time: 10 minutes

Nutrition Information Per Serving (1 serving unit):

Calories: 90, Carbohydrates: 17g, Saturated Fat: 0.1g, Protein: 3g, Fat: 1g, Sodium: 200mg, Potassium: 120mg, Fiber: 3g, Sugar: 2g, Vitamin C: 1.2mg, Calcium: 22mg, Iron: 0.8mg

Ingredients:

- 2 sheets nori seaweed
- 1/2 cup cooked short-grain brown rice, cooled
- 1/4 cucumber, julienned
- 1/4 carrot, julienned
- 1/4 red bell pepper, julienned
- 1/4 avocado, thinly sliced
- 1 tablespoon rice vinegar
- 1 teaspoon low-sodium soy sauce
- Optional: a pinch of sesame seeds for garnish

Directions:

1. Lay a nori sheet on a bamboo sushi mat or a piece of parchment paper.
2. Spread half of the cooked brown rice evenly onto the nori, leaving about an inch of space at the top.
3. Drizzle the rice with rice vinegar and low-sodium soy sauce.
4. Place half of the julienned cucumber, carrot, red bell pepper, and avocado slices in a line along the bottom third of the rice-covered nori.
5. Carefully roll the nori over the filling, using the mat or paper to help create a tight roll. Seal the edge with a little water if needed.
6. Repeat with the second sheet of nori and the remaining ingredients.

7. With a sharp knife, slice each roll into six pieces.

8. Serve the Veggie Nori Rolls with an optional sprinkle of sesame seeds on top.

20. Baked Kale Chips

⏰ **Time:** 30 minutes	🍽 **Serving Size:** 4 bowls
⚖ **Prep Time:** 10 minutes	👨‍🍳 **Cook Time:** 20 minutes

Nutrition Information Per Serving (1 serving bowl):

Calories: 50, Carbohydrates: 10g, Saturated Fat: 0g, Protein: 3g, Fat: 1g, Sodium: 30mg, Potassium: 299mg, Fiber: 2g, Sugar: 0g, Vitamin C: 19.2mg, Calcium: 53mg, Iron: 1mg

Ingredients:

- 1 bunch of kale, washed and dried
- 1 tablespoon olive oil
- 1/4 teaspoon salt (optional)

Directions:

1. Preheat your oven to 300°F.

2. Tear the kale leaves into bite-sized pieces after removing them from their thick stalks.

3. In a large bowl, gently toss the kale pieces with olive oil and salt, if using, until evenly coated.

4. Arrange the kale in a single layer on a baking sheet lined with parchment paper.

5. Bake for ten minutes in a preheated oven, then flip the leaves over and continue baking for an additional ten minutes, or until the edges are browned but not burned.

6. Allow the kale chips to cool slightly before serving. Enjoy this crunchy, nutritious snack!

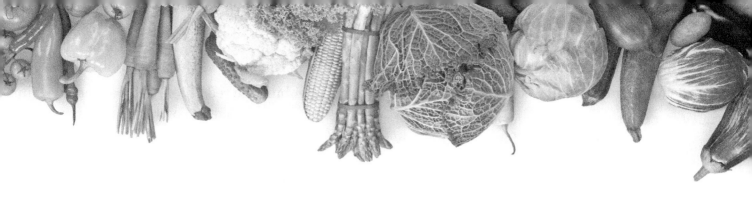

CHAPTER 4: BASIC RECIPES

21. Basic Quinoa

⏰ **Time:** 25 minutes	🍽 **Serving Size:** 4 bowls
⚖ **Prep Time:** 5 minutes	👨‍🍳 **Cook Time:** 20 minutes

Nutrition Information Per Serving (1 serving bowl):

Calories: 156, Carbohydrates: 27g, Saturated Fat: 0g, Protein: 6g, Fat: 2.5g, Sodium: 13mg, Potassium: 239mg, Fiber: 3g, Sugar: 0g, Vitamin C: 0mg, Calcium: 20mg, Iron: 2mg

Ingredients:

- 1 cup quinoa
- Pinch of salt (optional)
- 2 cups water or low-sodium chicken broth

Directions:

1. To get rid of the saponin, the quinoa's natural covering that can give it an unpleasant or soapy taste, rinse it under cold running water.

2. In a medium-sized pot, combine the rinsed quinoa, water or broth, and a pinch of salt if desired.

3. Over medium-high heat, bring the mixture to a boil. After that, lower the heat to a simmer, cover, and let the quinoa cook for 15 to 20 minutes, or until the liquid is absorbed and the quinoa is fluffy.

4. Remove the pot from heat and let it stand covered for 5 minutes. Fluff the quinoa gently with a fork before serving.

5. Serve as a base for salads, as a side dish, or use in other recipes that call for cooked grains.

22. Steamed Brown Rice

⏰ **Time:** 50 minutes	🍽 **Serving Size:** 4 bowls
⚖ **Prep Time:** 5 minutes	👨‍🍳 **Cook Time:** 45 minutes

Nutrition Information Per Serving (1 serving bowl):

Calories: 216, Carbohydrates: 45g, Saturated Fat: 0g, Protein: 5g, Fat: 1.6g, Sodium: 10mg, Potassium: 154mg, Fiber: 3.5g, Sugar: 0g, Vitamin C: 0mg, Calcium: 20mg, Iron: 1mg

Ingredients:

- 1 cup brown rice
- 2 cups water
- 1/4 teaspoon salt (optional)

Directions:

1. Rinse the brown rice under cold water using a fine mesh strainer until the water runs clear.

2. Rinse the rice and place it in a medium pot with a tight-fitting lid. Add water and salt to taste.

3. Bring the mixture to a boil over high heat.

4. After the rice starts to boil, lower the heat to a simmer, cover, and cook for approximately 45 minutes, or until the rice is soft and the water has been absorbed.

5. Take the rice off of the heat source and leave it covered for five minutes so that it can continue to steam and get fluffier.

6. Before serving, use a fork to fluff the rice.

23. Oven-Roasted Vegetables

⏰ Time: 45 minutes	🍽 Serving Size: 4
⚖ Prep Time: 15 minutes	👨‍🍳 Cook Time: 30 minutes

Nutrition Information Per Serving (1 cup):

Calories: 118, Carbohydrates: 25g, Saturated Fat: 0.4g, Protein: 4g, Fat: 0.2g, Sodium: 58mg, Potassium: 771mg, Fiber: 6g, Sugar: 9g, Vitamin C: 77mg, Calcium: 48mg, Iron: 1.4mg

Ingredients:

- 2 medium carrots, peeled and sliced
- 1 bell pepper, any color, seeded and chopped
- 1 zucchini, sliced into half-moons
- 1 yellow squash, sliced into half-moons
- 1 small red onion, cut into wedges
- 2 tablespoons balsamic vinegar
- Salt and pepper to taste (optional)
- Fresh herbs (such as thyme or rosemary), finely chopped (optional)

Directions:

1. Preheat your oven to 425°F (220°C).

2. Wash the vegetables and cut them into uniform pieces so that they cook evenly.

3. Combine the red onion, bell pepper, zucchini, yellow squash, and carrots in a big bowl and toss them with the balsamic vinegar. If preferred, add salt and pepper for seasoning.

4. Arrange the vegetables in a single layer on a parchment paper-lined baking sheet.

5. Roast, tossing occasionally, in the preheated oven for 25 to 30 minutes, or until the veggies are soft and beginning to caramelize.

6. If desired, sprinkle with fresh herbs before serving for added flavor.

7. Serve warm as an accompaniment to salads or wraps, or let cool and serve cold.

24. Grilled Tofu Steaks

⏰ Time: 25 minutes	🍽 Serving Size: 4 steaks
⚖ Prep Time: 10 minutes	👨‍🍳 Cook Time: 15 minutes

Nutrition Information Per Serving (1 steak):

Calories: 150, Carbohydrates: 4g, Saturated Fat: 0.5g, Protein: 16g, Fat: 8g, Sodium: 15mg, Potassium: 300mg, Fiber: 1g, Sugar: 1g, Vitamin C: 0mg, Calcium: 680mg, Iron: 2.9mg

Ingredients:

- 14 oz block of extra-firm tofu
- 2 tablespoons low-sodium soy sauce
- 1 tablespoon olive oil
- 1 teaspoon garlic powder
- 1 teaspoon onion powder
- Fresh ground black pepper to taste
- Non-stick cooking spray (for grilling)

Directions:

1. After draining, press the tofu between paper towels to remove as much moisture as you can.

2. Slice the tofu into four equal-sized steaks.

3. Mix the olive oil, black pepper, onion powder, garlic powder, and low-sodium soy sauce in a small bowl.

4. Marinate the tofu steaks in the mixture for at least 10 minutes, turning them occasionally to coat evenly.

5. Preheat your grill or grill pan over medium heat and coat it with non-stick cooking spray.

6. After placing the tofu steaks on the grill, cook them for 7 to 8 minutes on each side, or until they are thoroughly heated and have excellent grill marks.

7. Serve the grilled tofu steaks hot, garnished with fresh herbs if desired.

25. Simple Marinara Sauce

⏰ **Time:** 40 minutes	🍽 **Serving Size:** 6
⚖ **Prep Time:** 5 minutes	👨‍🍳 **Cook Time:** 35 minutes

Nutrition Information Per Serving (1 serving unit):

Calories: 90, Carbohydrates: 13g, Saturated Fat: 0g, Protein: 2g, Fat: 4g, Sodium: 300mg, Potassium: 364mg, Fiber: 3g, Sugar: 8g, Vitamin C: 20mg, Calcium: 30mg, Iron: 1mg

Ingredients:

- 1 tablespoon olive oil
- 1 small onion, finely chopped
- 2 garlic cloves, minced
- 1 can (28 ounces) crushed tomatoes
- 1 teaspoon dried basil
- 1 teaspoon dried oregano
- 1/2 teaspoon salt
- 1/4 teaspoon black pepper
- 1/2 teaspoon sugar (optional)
- Fresh basil leaves for garnish (optional)

Directions:

1. In a big saucepan, warm the olive oil over medium heat.

2. Add the finely chopped onion and cook until translucent, about 5 minutes.

3. Add the minced garlic and stir. Cook for one more minute, or until fragrant.

4. Add the smashed tomatoes, salt, black pepper, dried oregano, and dried basil.

5. If desired, add sugar to balance the acidity of the tomatoes.

6. After bringing the sauce to a simmer, lower the heat to low and simmer it, covered, for thirty minutes, stirring now and then.

7. Taste and adjust seasoning if necessary.

8. Serve hot over cooked pasta, or use as a base for other dishes. Garnish with fresh basil leaves if desired.

26. Roasted Butternut Squash Soup

⏰ **Time:** 55 minutes	🍽 **Serving Size:** 4 bowls
⚖ **Prep Time:** 15 minutes	👨‍🍳 **Cook Time:** 40 minutes

Nutrition Information Per Serving (1 bowl):

Calories: 175, Carbohydrates: 30g, Saturated Fat: 1g, Protein: 3g, Fat: 7g, Sodium: 480mg, Potassium: 670mg, Fiber: 5g, Sugar: 6g, Vitamin C: 31mg, Calcium: 100mg, Iron: 1.2mg

Ingredients:

- 1 medium butternut squash (about 2 pounds), peeled, seeded, and cut into 1-inch cubes
- 2 tablespoons olive oil
- 1/4 teaspoon salt
- 1/4 teaspoon ground black pepper
- 4 cups low-sodium vegetable broth
- 1 medium onion, chopped
- 2 garlic cloves, minced
- 1/2 teaspoon dried thyme
- 1/4 teaspoon ground nutmeg
- Optional garnish: chopped parsley or chives

Directions:

1. Set the oven's temperature to 400°F.

2. On a baking sheet, toss the butternut squash cubes with olive oil, salt, and black pepper.

3. Roast, stirring halfway through, in a preheated oven for 25 minutes, or until the squash is soft and gently browned.

4. Preheat a big saucepan over medium heat while the squash roasts. After adding the last tablespoon of olive oil, sauté the onion for five minutes or until it becomes transparent.

5. Cook for a further minute or until aromatic after adding the ground nutmeg, dry thyme, and chopped garlic to the onions.

6. Include the low-sodium vegetable broth in the pot with the roasted butternut squash.

7. Simmer the mixture for 15 minutes to give the flavors time to blend.

8. Puree the soup with an immersion blender until it's smooth. In case you don't own an immersion blender, cautiously move the soup into batches and process it in a blender till it becomes smooth.

9. Transfer the soup back to the pot to fully reheat, taste and adjust the spice, and serve hot, topped with chopped parsley or chives, if preferred.

27. Steamed Green Beans with Lemon Zest

⏰	**Time:** 25 minutes	🍽️	**Serving Size:** 4
⚖️	**Prep Time:** 5 minutes	👨‍🍳	**Cook Time:** 20 minutes

Nutrition Information Per Serving (1 cup):

Calories: 40, Carbohydrates: 9g, Saturated Fat: 0g, Protein: 2g, Fat: 0.1g, Sodium: 6mg, Potassium: 230mg, Fiber: 4g, Sugar: 2g, Vitamin C: 12.2mg, Calcium: 41mg, Iron: 1mg

Ingredients:

- 1 pound fresh green beans, ends trimmed
- Zest of 1 lemon
- Juice of 1/2 lemon
- 1 teaspoon olive oil (optional)
- Salt and pepper to taste (optional)

Directions:

1. Add two inches or so of water to a pot and bring it to a boil.

2. Fill a steamer basket with green beans, then place the basket over a pot of boiling water. Make sure the steamer basket's bottom is not in contact with the water.

3. Place a lid on the saucepan and steam the green beans for ten to fifteen minutes, or until they are soft enough for your taste.

4. After the green beans are steam-cooked, move them to a bowl for serving.

5. Squeeze the lemon juice and finely grate the zest of the lemon over the green beans.

6. Season with salt and pepper to taste and sprinkle with a teaspoon of olive oil, if desired.

7. Toss the green beans to spread the spice, zest, and juice of the lemon equally.

8. Serve the steaming green beans as a crisp and energizing side dish.

28. Baked Sweet Potatoes

⏰ **Time:** 1 hour	🍽 **Serving Size:** 4 potatoes
⚖ **Prep Time:** 5 minutes	👨‍🍳 **Cook Time:** 55 minutes

Nutrition Information Per Serving (1 potatoe):

Calories: 162, Carbohydrates: 37g, Saturated Fat: 0.1g, Protein: 2g, Fat: 0.2g, Sodium: 72mg, Potassium: 542mg, Fiber: 5g, Sugar: 12g, Vitamin C: 3.1mg, Calcium: 52mg, Iron: 1.1mg

Ingredients:

- 4 medium sweet potatoes, scrubbed clean

- Optional toppings: a sprinkle of cinnamon, a dollop of unsweetened applesauce, or a drizzle of honey (for those who can tolerate a small amount of sugar)

Directions:

1. Set the oven's temperature to 400°F.

2. Using a fork, pierce the sweet potatoes all over to let steam escape while they cook.

3. For easier cleanup, put the sweet potatoes on a baking sheet covered with parchment paper or aluminum foil.

4. Bake for about 55 minutes, or until a fork inserted into the sweet potatoes comes out soft.

5. Before serving, take the sweet potatoes out of the oven and allow them to cool somewhat.

6. Before serving, if preferred, split the sweet potatoes open and top with any of the optional ingredients.

29. Cilantro Lime Rice

⏰ **Time:** 35 minutes	🍽 **Serving Size:** 4 cups
⚖ **Prep Time:** 5 minutes	👨‍🍳 **Cook Time:** 30 minutes

Nutrition Information Per Serving (1 cup):

Calories: 200, Carbohydrates: 45g, Saturated Fat: 0.5g, Protein: 4g, Fat: 1g, Sodium: 10mg, Potassium: 55mg, Fiber: 0.6g, Sugar: 0.1g, Vitamin C: 2.5mg, Calcium: 16mg, Iron: 0.4mg

Ingredients:

- 1 cup long-grain white rice
- 2 cups water
- 1/2 teaspoon salt
- 1 lime, zest and juice
- 1/4 cup fresh cilantro, chopped

Directions:

1. To get rid of extra starch, rinse the rice in cold water until the water flows clear.

2. Place the washed rice, water, and salt in a medium pot. Bring over high heat to a boil.

3. After the rice starts to boil, lower the heat to a simmer, cover, and cook for eighteen minutes, or until the water is absorbed and the rice is soft.

4. Take the pot off of the burner and leave it covered for five minutes so the rice can steam.

5. Use a fork to separate the grains in the rice. Add the fresh cilantro, lime juice, and zest and stir until thoroughly mixed.

6. As a tasty side dish, serve warm cilantro lime rice.

30. Homemade Vegetable Broth

⏰ **Time:** 1 hour	🍽 **Serving Size:** 6 cups
⚖ **Prep Time:** 10 minutes	👨‍🍳 **Cook Time:** 50 minutes

Nutrition Information Per Serving (1 cup):

Calories: 15, Carbohydrates: 3g, Saturated Fat: 0g, Protein: 0g, Fat: 0g, Sodium: 150mg, Potassium: 60mg, Fiber: 1g, Sugar: 2g, Vitamin C: 2mg, Calcium: 20mg, Iron: 0.4mg

Ingredients:

- 2 carrots, chopped
- 2 stalks of celery, chopped
- 1 large onion, chopped
- 4 cloves of garlic, minced
- 1 bay leaf
- A small bunch of fresh parsley
- A few sprigs of fresh thyme
- 1 teaspoon of salt (optional)
- 8 cups of water

Directions:

1. Prepare your vegetables by washing and roughly chopping the carrots, celery, and onion. Peel and mince the garlic.

2. In a large pot, combine the chopped vegetables, garlic, bay leaf, parsley, thyme, and salt if using.

3. Fill the pot with the eight glasses of water. Over high heat, bring the mixture to a boil.

4. Once boiling, reduce the heat to low and let the broth simmer, uncovered, for about 50 minutes. The longer it simmers, the more flavorful it will be.

5. Once the broth has reached a simmer, pour it through a fine-mesh sieve into a big basin or pot and dispose of the particles.

6. Let the broth cool before putting it in storage containers. You can store the broth in the fridge for up to a week or freeze it for up to three months.

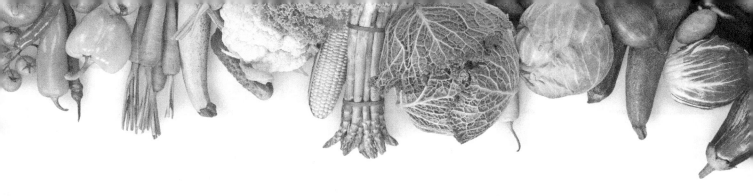

CHAPTER 5: VEGAN AND VEGETARIAN

31. Stuffed Bell Peppers with Quinoa

	Time: 55 minutes		Serving Size: 4 peppers
	Prep Time: 15 minutes		Cook Time: 40 minutes

Nutrition Information Per Serving (1 stuffed pepper):

Calories: 265, Carbohydrates: 50g, Saturated Fat: 0.5g, Protein: 9g, Fat: 3g, Sodium: 15mg, Potassium: 451mg, Fiber: 7g, Sugar: 6g, Vitamin C: 169mg, Calcium: 34mg, Iron: 2.7mg

Ingredients:

- 4 large bell peppers, any color
- 1 cup quinoa, rinsed
- 2 cups vegetable broth
- 1 medium onion, diced
- 2 cloves garlic, minced
- 1 zucchini, diced
- 1 cup fresh spinach, chopped
- 1 teaspoon olive oil
- 1/2 teaspoon ground cumin
- 1/2 teaspoon paprika
- Salt and pepper to taste
- Fresh parsley, for garnish

Directions:

1. Set the oven's temperature to 375°F.

2. Cut the bell peppers' tops off, removing the seeds and membranes. Put aside.

3. Bring the vegetable broth to a boil in a medium saucepan. Reduce heat to low, cover, and add quinoa. Simmer for fifteen minutes, or until the quinoa is soft and the broth has been absorbed.

4. In a skillet over medium heat, warm the olive oil while the quinoa cooks. Add the onion and garlic and sauté for about 3 minutes, or until transparent.

5. Cook the zucchini for a further five minutes after adding it to the skillet. Add the spinach and simmer, stirring, until it wilts.

6. After the quinoa is cooked, add it to the skillet with the vegetables and fluff it with a fork. Add the paprika and cumin, then season to taste with salt and pepper.

7. Tightly pack the quinoa and veggie mixture into each bell pepper.

8. Transfer the filled peppers to a baking tray and bake for 20 minutes, or until the peppers are soft, in a preheated oven.

9. Before serving, garnish with fresh parsley.

32. Vegan Chili with Sweet Potato

⏰ **Time:** 1 hour	🍽 **Serving Size:** 6 potatoes
⚖ **Prep Time:** 15 minutes	👨‍🍳 **Cook Time:** 45 minutes

Nutrition Information Per Serving (1 cup):

Calories: 290, Carbohydrates: 54g, Saturated Fat: 0.5g, Protein: 12g, Fat: 3g, Sodium: 480mg, Potassium: 900mg, Fiber: 14g, Sugar: 13g, Vitamin C: 25mg, Calcium: 80mg, Iron: 4mg

Ingredients:

- 2 medium sweet potatoes, peeled and cubed
- 1 tablespoon olive oil
- 1 large onion, chopped
- 3 cloves garlic, minced
- 1 bell pepper, diced
- 1 can (15 ounces) black beans, drained and rinsed
- 1 can (15 ounces) kidney beans, drained and rinsed
- 1 can (28 ounces) diced tomatoes
- 3 tablespoons tomato paste
- 2 cups vegetable broth
- 1 tablespoon chili powder
- 1 teaspoon ground cumin
- 1 teaspoon smoked paprika
- 1/2 teaspoon ground cinnamon
- Salt and pepper to taste
- Fresh cilantro, for garnish

Directions:

1. Heat the olive oil in a big pot over medium heat. Add the onion and garlic, and cook for about 5 minutes, or until the onion is tender and transparent.

2. Cook the sweet potatoes and bell pepper in the pot for a further five minutes, stirring now and then.

3. Add the chili powder, cumin, smoked paprika, diced tomatoes, kidney beans, tomato paste, vegetable broth, and cinnamon. To taste, add salt and pepper for seasoning.

4. Once the sweet potatoes are soft, bring the chili to a boil, lower the heat, and simmer it covered for 30 minutes.

5. Garnish the hot chili with fresh cilantro. Have fun!

33. Eggplant Parmesan Casserole

⏰ **Time:** 1 hour 10 min	🍽 **Serving Size:** 6
⚖ **Prep Time:** 20 minutes	👨‍🍳 **Cook Time:** 50 minutes

Nutrition Information Per Serving (1 serving):

Calories: 230, Carbohydrates: 35g, Saturated Fat: 1g, Protein: 8g, Fat: 7g, Sodium: 320mg, Potassium: 717mg, Fiber: 11g, Sugar: 13g, Vitamin C: 12mg, Calcium: 130mg, Iron: 2mg

Ingredients:

- 2 large eggplants, sliced into 1/2-inch rounds
- 3 cups marinara sauce, low sodium
- 1 cup vegan mozzarella cheese, shredded
- 1/2 cup fresh basil leaves, chopped
- 2 tablespoons nutritional yeast
- 1 tablespoon olive oil
- 1 teaspoon garlic powder
- 1 teaspoon dried oregano
- Salt and pepper to taste
- Cooking spray

Directions:

1. Set the oven's temperature to 375°F.

2. To extract moisture, sprinkle the eggplant slices with salt and allow them to sit for approximately ten minutes. Using paper towels, pat dry.

3. Spread cooking spray on a baking sheet and line it with slices of eggplant, arranging them in a single layer. Bake, rotating them midway through, until they are soft and beginning to turn golden, about 20 minutes.

4. Combine the nutritional yeast, dried oregano, garlic powder, salt, and pepper in a small bowl.

5. Apply a thin layer of marinara sauce to a casserole dish.

6. Cover the sauce with a layer of cooked eggplant pieces. Add half of the chopped basil and the nutritional yeast mixture on top.

7. Top with half of the vegan mozzarella cheese and another layer of marinara sauce.

8. Continue layering the eggplant until all of it is utilized, and then top with a layer of marinara sauce and the leftover vegan mozzarella cheese.

9. Brush with olive oil and bake for 30 minutes in a preheated oven, or until the cheese is bubbling and melted.

10. Before serving, garnish with the remaining fresh basil.

34. Tofu Scramble with Vegetables

⏰ **Time:** 30 minutes	🍽 **Serving Size:** 4
⚖ **Prep Time:** 10 minutes	👨‍🍳 **Cook Time:** 20 minutes

Nutrition Information Per Serving (1 serving unit):

Calories: 150, Carbohydrates: 10g, Saturated Fat: 1g, Protein: 14g, Fat: 8g, Sodium: 200mg, Potassium: 300mg, Fiber: 3g, Sugar: 4g, Vitamin C: 20mg, Calcium: 150mg, Iron: 2.5mg

Ingredients:

- 14 oz firm tofu, drained and crumbled
- 1 tablespoon olive oil
- 1/2 teaspoon turmeric
- 1/4 teaspoon black salt (kala namak), optional for eggy flavor
- 1 small onion, diced
- 1 bell pepper, diced
- 1 cup spinach, chopped
- 1/2 cup cherry tomatoes, halved
- 1/4 cup nutritional yeast
- Salt and pepper to taste
- Fresh parsley, chopped, for garnish

Directions:

1. In a large, nonstick skillet, heat the olive oil over medium heat. Add the bell peppers and onions, and sauté for approximately 5 minutes, or until the peppers are soft and the onions are transparent.

2. Crumble the tofu into the skillet and top it with black salt and turmeric. After combining everything, simmer for a further five minutes, letting the tofu get a little brown.

3. Cook the spinach in the skillet for about two minutes, or until it has wilted, along with the cherry tomatoes.

4. Add the nutritional yeast and season with the pepper and salt. Cook for another three minutes, stirring now and then.

5. Before serving, garnish with fresh parsley. Enjoy your wholesome tofu scramble with veggies while it's still hot.

35. Butternut Squash and Black Bean Enchiladas

⏰ **Time:** 1 hour	🍽️ **Serving Size:** 6 enchiladas
⚖️ **Prep Time:** 20 minutes	👨‍🍳 **Cook Time:** 40 minutes

Nutrition Information Per Serving (1 enchilada):

Calories: 250, Carbohydrates: 45g, Saturated Fat: 1g, Protein: 8g, Fat: 3.5g, Sodium: 350mg, Potassium: 670mg, Fiber: 9g, Sugar: 5g, Vitamin C: 20mg, Calcium: 50mg, Iron: 3mg

Ingredients:

- 1 medium butternut squash, peeled and cubed
- 1 can (15 ounces) black beans, drained and rinsed
- 1 medium onion, diced
- 2 cloves garlic, minced
- 1 teaspoon ground cumin
- 1/2 teaspoon chili powder
- 1/2 teaspoon smoked paprika
- Salt and pepper to taste
- 8 whole wheat tortillas
- 2 cups red enchilada sauce, low-fat
- 1/4 cup fresh cilantro, chopped
- Cooking spray

Directions:

1. Set the oven's temperature to 375°F.
2. Transfer the cubed butternut squash to a baking sheet, sprinkle with salt and pepper, and give it a quick coat of cooking spray. Roast until soft, about 25 minutes.
3. Put the black beans, smoked paprika, cumin, chili powder, onion, and garlic in a big bowl along with the roasted butternut squash. To taste, add more salt or pepper.
4. Fill a baking dish with 1/2 cup of enchilada sauce and cover with cooking spray.
5. Tightly roll each tortilla after stuffing it with the squash and bean mixture, then put it seam side down in the baking dish.
6. Ensure that all of the rolled tortillas are covered with the remaining enchilada sauce.
7. Bake the baking dish for fifteen minutes with the foil covering it.
8. Take off the foil and continue baking for a further five minutes, or until the sauce begins to bubble.
9. Before serving, garnish with fresh cilantro.

36. Cauliflower Steak with Herb Sauce

⏰ **Time:** 45 minutes	🍽️ **Serving Size:** 4 steaks
⚖️ **Prep Time:** 15 minutes	👨‍🍳 **Cook Time:** 30 minutes

Nutrition Information Per Serving (1 steak):

Calories: 180, Carbohydrates: 14g, Saturated Fat: 1g, Protein: 5g, Fat: 12g, Sodium: 150mg, Potassium: 446mg, Fiber: 5g, Sugar: 5g, Vitamin C: 69mg, Calcium: 32mg, Iron: 1mg

Ingredients:

- 1 large head of cauliflower
- 2 tablespoons olive oil
- 1/2 teaspoon garlic powder
- Salt and pepper to taste
- 1/4 cup fresh parsley, finely chopped
- 2 tablespoons fresh chives, finely chopped
- 1 tablespoon fresh tarragon, finely chopped
- 1 tablespoon fresh lemon juice
- 1 teaspoon lemon zest
- 1/4 cup low-sodium vegetable broth
- 1 tablespoon capers, rinsed and chopped

Directions:

1. Preheat the oven to 400°F.

2. Remove the leaves from the cauliflower and cut the head into 4 thick slices, creating 'steaks.'

3. Season each cauliflower steak on both sides with salt, pepper, and garlic powder after brushing it with olive oil.

4. After putting the cauliflower steaks on a baking sheet, roast them for about 30 minutes, turning them over halfway through, or until they are soft and golden brown.

5. While the cauliflower is roasting, prepare the herb sauce by combining parsley, chives, tarragon, lemon juice, lemon zest, vegetable broth, and capers in a small bowl.

6. Once the cauliflower steaks are done, transfer them to serving plates.

7. Spoon the herb sauce over the cauliflower steaks and serve immediately.

37. Zucchini Noodles with Avocado Pesto

⏱ **Time:** 25 minutes	🍽 **Serving Size:** 2 plates
⚖ **Prep Time:** 15 minutes	👨‍🍳 **Cook Time:** 10 minutes

Nutrition Information Per Serving (1 plate):

Calories: 320, Carbohydrates: 24g, Saturated Fat: 4g, Protein: 8g, Fat: 24g, Sodium: 210mg, Potassium: 1020mg, Fiber: 10g, Sugar: 8g, Vitamin C: 35mg, Calcium: 50mg, Iron: 2mg

Ingredients:

- 2 medium zucchinis
- 1 ripe avocado
- 1/2 cup fresh basil leaves
- 2 cloves garlic
- 2 tablespoons pine nuts
- 2 tablespoons lemon juice
- 1/4 teaspoon salt
- 1/4 teaspoon black pepper
- 1 tablespoon nutritional yeast (optional for a cheesy flavor)
- 2 tablespoons extra-virgin olive oil
- Cherry tomatoes for garnish (optional)

Directions:

1. Spiralise the zucchini to make noodles, then set aside.

2. Put the avocado, pine nuts, garlic, basil leaves, lemon juice, salt, pepper, and nutritional yeast—if using—in a food processor. Process till smooth.

3. Slowly pour in the olive oil while the food processor is operating, until the pesto has a creamy consistency.

4. Toss the zucchini noodles with the avocado pesto in a big bowl until evenly coated.

5. If wanted, top right now with cherry tomatoes and serve.

38. Sweet Potato and Chickpea Stew

⏱ **Time:** 50 minutes	🍽 **Serving Size:** 4 bowls
⚖ **Prep Time:** 10 minutes	👨‍🍳 **Cook Time:** 40 minutes

Nutrition Information Per Serving (1 bowl):

Calories: 260, Carbohydrates: 45g, Saturated Fat: 1g, Protein: 7g, Fat: 5g, Sodium: 300mg, Potassium: 670mg, Fiber: 9g, Sugar: 13g, Vitamin C: 5mg, Calcium: 80mg, Iron: 3mg

Ingredients:

- 2 medium sweet potatoes, peeled and cubed
- 1 can (15 ounces) chickpeas, drained and rinsed
- 1 tablespoon olive oil
- 1 large onion, diced
- 2 cloves garlic, minced
- 1 teaspoon ground cumin
- 1/2 teaspoon ground coriander
- 1/2 teaspoon smoked paprika
- 1/4 teaspoon cayenne pepper (optional)
- 4 cups low-sodium vegetable broth
- 1 can (14.5 ounces) diced tomatoes, no-salt-added
- 2 cups baby spinach leaves
- Salt and pepper to taste
- Fresh cilantro, chopped (for garnish)

Directions:

1. Heat the olive oil in a large pot over medium heat. Add the onion and garlic, sautéing until the onion is translucent, about 5 minutes.

2. Stir in the ground cumin, coriander, smoked paprika, and cayenne pepper, cooking for another minute until fragrant.

3. Add the diced tomatoes, chickpeas, sweet potatoes, and vegetable broth to the pot. Once the mixture reaches a boil, reduce the heat and cook the sweet potatoes until they are tender, about 30 minutes.

4. Add the baby spinach and cook, stirring, until the spinach wilts, about 2 minutes. Adjust the seasoning with salt and pepper to taste.

5. Serve the stew garnished with fresh cilantro.

39. Vegan Shepherd's Pie

Time: 1 hour	**Serving Size:** 6
Prep Time: 20 minutes	**Cook Time:** 40 minutes

Nutrition Information Per Serving (1 serving unit):

Calories: 275, Carbohydrates: 49g, Saturated Fat: 1g, Protein: 9g, Fat: 5g, Sodium: 320mg, Potassium: 811mg, Fiber: 11g, Sugar: 8g, Vitamin C: 22mg, Calcium: 55mg, Iron: 3mg

Ingredients:

- 2 lbs sweet potatoes, peeled and cubed
- 1 tablespoon olive oil
- 1 medium onion, diced
- 2 cloves garlic, minced
- 1 carrot, diced
- 1 celery stalk, diced
- 1 cup brown lentils, rinsed and drained
- 3 cups low-sodium vegetable broth
- 1 teaspoon dried thyme
- 1 teaspoon dried rosemary
- 1/2 teaspoon paprika
- Salt and pepper to taste
- 1 cup frozen peas
- 1 cup frozen corn
- 1/4 cup unsweetened almond milk
- 1 tablespoon vegan butter

Directions:

1. Set the oven's temperature to 400°F.

2. Put the sweet potatoes in a big pot and add water to cover. After bringing to a boil, lower the heat and simmer for 15 minutes or until the food is soft.

3. In a big skillet set over medium heat, warm up the olive oil while the sweet potatoes are cooking. Sauté the garlic and onion until transparent.

4. Cook the celery and carrot in the skillet for five minutes, or until they are tender.

5. Add the lentils, salt, pepper, paprika, rosemary, thyme, and vegetable broth. Once the lentils are soft, bring to a boil, then lower the heat and simmer for 25 minutes.

6. Cook for a further five minutes after adding the frozen peas and corn to the lentil mixture.

7. After draining, mash the sweet potatoes until smooth, adding almond milk and vegan butter as needed. To taste, add salt and pepper for seasoning.

8. Transfer the lentil mixture onto an ovenproof dish and cover with the mashed sweet potatoes.

9. Bake for 20 minutes, or until the top is beginning to turn brown, in a preheated oven.

10. Before serving, let the shepherd's pie cool for a few minutes.

40. Stuffed Acorn Squash

⏰ Time: 1 hour 10 min	🍽 Serving Size: 4
⚖ Prep Time: 15 minutes	👨‍🍳 Cook Time: 55 minutes

Nutrition Information Per Serving (1 serving unit):

Calories: 298, Carbohydrates: 67g, Saturated Fat: 1g, Protein: 6g, Fat: 3g, Sodium: 202mg, Potassium: 1345mg, Fiber: 11g, Sugar: 5g, Vitamin C: 40mg, Calcium: 109mg, Iron: 3mg

Ingredients:

- 2 acorn squashes, halved and seeds removed
- 1 cup quinoa, rinsed
- 2 cups low-sodium vegetable broth
- 1 small red onion, diced
- 1 red bell pepper, diced
- 2 cloves garlic, minced
- 1 cup kale, chopped
- 1 teaspoon dried thyme
- 1 teaspoon dried rosemary
- Salt and pepper to taste
- Fresh parsley, chopped (for garnish)

Directions:

1. Preheat the oven to 400°F.

2. After placing the halves of the acorn squash cut-side up on a baking sheet, bake for 40 minutes, or until the squash is fork-tender.

3. While the squash is baking, cook the quinoa in the vegetable broth according to package instructions, usually about 15 minutes.

4. Add the onion, bell pepper, and garlic to a skillet over medium heat and sauté for about 5 minutes, or until the onion becomes transparent.

5. Add the kale, thyme, rosemary, and cooked quinoa to the skillet. Stir to combine and cook for an additional 2 minutes. Season with salt and pepper.

6. Once the squash halves are baked, remove them from the oven and fill each half with the quinoa mixture.

7. Return the stuffed squashes to the oven and bake for an additional 15 minutes.

8. Garnish with fresh parsley before serving.

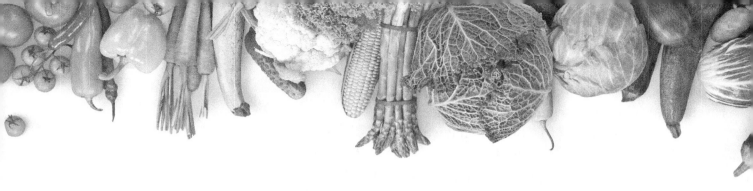

CHAPTER 6: SOUPS & STEWS

41. Carrot and Ginger Soup

⏰ Time: 50 minutes	🍽 Serving Size: 4 bowls
⚖ Prep Time: 10 minutes	👨‍🍳 Cook Time: 40 minutes

Nutrition Information Per Serving (1 bowl):

Calories: 120, Carbohydrates: 27g, Saturated Fat: 0.5g, Protein: 2g, Fat: 1g, Sodium: 150mg, Potassium: 689mg, Fiber: 6g, Sugar: 12g, Vitamin C: 10mg, Calcium: 48mg, Iron: 0.7mg

Ingredients:

- 1 tablespoon olive oil
- 4 cups chopped carrots
- 1 large onion, diced
- 3 cloves garlic, minced
- 2 tablespoons grated fresh ginger
- 4 cups low-sodium vegetable broth
- Salt and pepper to taste
- Fresh parsley for garnish (optional)

Directions:

1. Heat the olive oil in a big pot over medium heat. Add the onions and cook for about 5 minutes, or until they are transparent.

2. Cook the garlic and ginger in the pot for an additional two minutes, stirring often to avoid burning.

3. Add the chopped carrots and simmer, stirring, until they begin to soften, about 5 minutes.

4. Add the veggie broth and heat the blend until it boils. After the pot reaches a boil, lower the heat to a simmer and cover it. Cook until the carrots are extremely soft, about 30 minutes.

5. Puree the soup with an immersion blender until it's smooth. Should you not possess an immersion blender, cautiously move the soup in portions to a blender for smooth pureeing.

6. Add salt and pepper to taste when preparing the soup.

7. If preferred, top hot dish with freshly chopped parsley.

42. Chicken and Rice Soup

⏰ Time: 50 minutes	🍽 Serving Size: 4 bowls
⚖ Prep Time: 10 minutes	👨‍🍳 Cook Time: 40 minutes

Nutrition Information Per Serving (1 bowl):

Calories: 215, Carbohydrates: 28g, Saturated Fat: 1g, Protein: 18g, Fat: 4g, Sodium: 70mg, Potassium: 300mg, Fiber: 1g, Sugar: 3g, Vitamin C: 1mg, Calcium: 20mg, Iron: 1.5mg

Ingredients:

- 1/2 lb boneless, skinless chicken breasts
- 4 cups low-sodium chicken broth
- 1 cup cooked white rice
- 1 medium carrot, peeled and diced
- 1 celery stalk, diced
- 1 small onion, chopped
- 2 cloves garlic, minced
- 1/2 teaspoon dried thyme
- 1/2 teaspoon dried oregano
- Salt and pepper to taste
- 2 tablespoons chopped fresh parsley
- Lemon wedges for serving

Directions:

1. In a large pot, bring the chicken broth to a simmer over medium heat.

2. Add the chicken breasts to the pot and cook until no longer pink in the center, about 15 minutes. Remove the chicken, let cool slightly, and shred into bite-sized pieces.

3. Add the onion, celery, carrot, and garlic to the same saucepan. Cook for about 5 minutes, or until the vegetables are tender.

4. Return the shredded chicken to the pot and add the cooked rice, thyme, oregano, salt, and pepper. Simmer for another 20 minutes.

5. Add the fresh parsley just before serving.

6. Present the soup beside a wedge of lemon.

43. Tomato Basil Soup

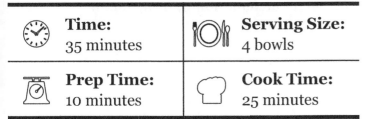

⏰ **Time:** 35 minutes	🍽 **Serving Size:** 4 bowls
⚖ **Prep Time:** 10 minutes	👨‍🍳 **Cook Time:** 25 minutes

Nutrition Information Per Serving (1 bowl):

Calories: 74, Carbohydrates: 16g, Saturated Fat: 0.1g, Protein: 2.7g, Fat: 0.4g, Sodium: 296mg, Potassium: 549mg, Fiber: 4g, Sugar: 9g, Vitamin C: 23mg, Calcium: 38mg, Iron: 0.9mg

Ingredients:

- 4 cups low-sodium vegetable broth
- 2 cans (14.5 ounces each) no-salt-added diced tomatoes
- 1 small onion, diced
- 2 cloves garlic, minced
- 1 carrot, peeled and diced
- 2 tablespoons fresh basil, chopped
- 1 teaspoon dried oregano
- Salt and pepper to taste
- Fresh basil leaves for garnish (optional)

Directions:

1. Place a little amount of water over medium heat in a big pot. Add the onions and garlic, and cook for about 5 minutes, or until the onions are transparent. As more water is required, add it to avoid sticking.

2. Cook the chopped carrot in the pot for a further three minutes.

3. Add the cans of diced tomatoes with juice and the veggie broth. Add the dried oregano and chopped basil and stir.

4. After bringing the soup to a boil, lower the heat, and simmer it until the veggies are soft, about 15 minutes.

5. Puree the soup in the pot directly with an immersion blender to the desired smoothness. If you don't have an immersion blender, you can alternatively carefully transfer the soup to a blender in batches.

6. Add salt and pepper to taste when preparing the soup.

7. If desired, top the heated soup with fresh basil leaves.

44. Vegetable Minestrone

	Time: 55 minutes		Serving Size: 4 bowls
	Prep Time: 15 minutes		Cook Time: 40 minutes

Nutrition Information Per Serving (1 bowl):

Calories: 190, Carbohydrates: 35g, Saturated Fat: 0.5g, Protein: 7g, Fat: 2g, Sodium: 210mg, Potassium: 600mg, Fiber: 8g, Sugar: 6g, Vitamin C: 18mg, Calcium: 60mg, Iron: 2.5mg

Ingredients:

- 1 tablespoon olive oil
- 1 small onion, diced
- 2 garlic cloves, minced
- 2 medium carrots, peeled and diced
- 1 zucchini, diced
- 1 yellow squash, diced
- 1/2 cup green beans, trimmed and cut into 1/2-inch pieces
- 4 cups low-sodium vegetable broth
- 2 cups water
- 1 (14.5-ounce) can no-salt-added diced tomatoes, with juice
- 1 teaspoon dried basil
- 1 teaspoon dried oregano
- 1/2 teaspoon dried thyme
- Salt and pepper to taste
- 1/2 cup uncooked small whole wheat pasta, such as shells or macaroni
- 1 (15-ounce) can low-sodium cannellini beans, drained and rinsed
- 2 cups fresh baby spinach leaves
- 1 tablespoon fresh lemon juice

Directions:

1. In a big pot over medium heat, warm the olive oil. Add the onion and garlic, and cook for about 5 minutes, or until the onion becomes transparent.

2. Add the green beans, zucchini, yellow squash, and carrots and stir. Simmer the vegetables for an additional five minutes, or until they begin to soften.

3. Add the water and veggie broth. Season with salt and pepper and add the diced tomatoes with their juice, basil, oregano, and thyme. Heat the mixture until it boils.

4. After it reaches a boiling point, lower the heat and simmer for 20 minutes.

5. Fill the saucepan with the pasta and cannellini beans. Simmer for a further 10 minutes or until the pasta is tender.

6. Add the spinach and simmer, stirring, for about 2 minutes, or until it wilts.

7. Turn off the heat and whisk in the lemon juice. If needed, adjust the seasoning by tasting it.

8. If wanted, top with freshly chopped parsley or basil and serve hot.

45. Pumpkin Soup with Coconut Milk

	Time: 1 hour		Serving Size: 4 bowls
	Prep Time: 15 minutes		Cook Time: 45 minutes

Nutrition Information Per Serving (1 bowl):

Calories: 180, Carbohydrates: 21g, Saturated Fat: 5g, Protein: 3g, Fat: 10g, Sodium: 150mg, Potassium: 470mg, Fiber: 5g, Sugar: 6g, Vitamin C: 9mg, Calcium: 30mg, Iron: 1.4mg

Ingredients:

- 2 cups pumpkin puree (fresh or canned without added sugar)
- 1 tablespoon olive oil
- 1 small onion, diced
- 2 garlic cloves, minced
- 3 cups low-sodium vegetable broth
- 1 cup light coconut milk
- 1/2 teaspoon ground ginger
- 1/4 teaspoon ground nutmeg
- Salt and pepper to taste
- Fresh parsley or cilantro for garnish (optional)

Directions:

1. In a large pot over medium heat, warm the olive oil. Add the chopped onion and simmer for 3–4 minutes, or until transparent.

2. Cook the minced garlic for a further minute, or until fragrant.

3. Add the ground nutmeg, ground ginger, vegetable broth, and pumpkin puree and stir. To taste, add salt and pepper for seasoning.

4. After bringing the mixture to a boil, lower the heat, and simmer it for 25 to 30 minutes while stirring now and again.

5. Add the light coconut milk and mix everything together. Simmer for a further ten to fifteen minutes.

6. Puree the soup with an immersion blender until it's smooth. In case you don't own an immersion blender, cautiously move the soup into batches and process it in a blender till it becomes smooth.

7. Garnish with cilantro or fresh parsley, if preferred, and serve hot.

46. Turkey and Vegetable Stew

⏱ **Time:** 1 hour 30 min	🍽 **Serving Size:** 6 bowls
⚖ **Prep Time:** 15 minutes	👨‍🍳 **Cook Time:** 1 hour 15 min

Nutrition Information Per Serving (1 bowl):

Calories: 250, Carbohydrates: 18g, Saturated Fat: 1g, Protein: 28g, Fat: 8g, Sodium: 420mg, Potassium: 740mg, Fiber: 4g, Sugar: 5g, Vitamin C: 25mg, Calcium: 50mg, Iron: 3mg

Ingredients:

- 1 lb turkey breast, cut into cubes
- 2 tablespoons olive oil
- 1 medium onion, diced
- 2 carrots, peeled and sliced
- 2 celery stalks, sliced
- 3 garlic cloves, minced
- 1 zucchini, diced
- 1 yellow squash, diced
- 1 can (14.5 oz) diced tomatoes, no salt added
- 4 cups low-sodium chicken broth
- 1 teaspoon dried thyme
- 1 teaspoon dried rosemary
- 1 bay leaf
- Salt and pepper to taste
- 2 cups spinach leaves, roughly chopped

Directions:

1. Heat the olive oil in a big pot over medium heat. After adding the turkey cubes, simmer for 5 to 7 minutes, or until browned all over. After taking the turkey out of the saucepan, set it aside.

2. Place the celery, carrots, and onion in the same saucepan. Sauté for approximately five minutes, or until the vegetables are tender. Once fragrant, add the garlic and simmer for an additional minute.

3. Add the diced tomatoes, yellow squash, and zucchini back to the pot with the turkey. Mix everything together.

4. Add the bay leaf, thyme, and rosemary to the chicken broth. After bringing to a boil, lower the heat to a simmer and cook for 60 minutes, or until the turkey is soft.

5. Season to taste with salt and pepper. Stir in the chopped spinach and heat until wilted, a few minutes before serving.

6. Before serving, take out the bay leaf. Enjoy your wholesome Turkey and Vegetable Stew while it's hot!

47. Pea and Ham Hock Soup

⏰ Time: 2 hours	🍽 Serving Size: 6 bowls
⚖ Prep Time: 20 minutes	👨‍🍳 Cook Time: 1 hour 40 min

Nutrition Information Per Serving (1 bowl):

Calories: 215, Carbohydrates: 20g, Saturated Fat: 1g, Protein: 25g, Fat: 4g, Sodium: 570mg, Potassium: 645mg, Fiber: 5g, Sugar: 4g, Vitamin C: 2mg, Calcium: 30mg, Iron: 2mg

Ingredients:

- 1 smoked ham hock (about 1 pound)
- 1 cup dried split peas
- 1 tablespoon olive oil
- 1 large carrot, diced
- 1 stalk celery, diced
- 1 small onion, diced
- 2 cloves garlic, minced
- 6 cups low-sodium chicken broth
- 1 bay leaf
- 1/2 teaspoon dried thyme
- Salt and pepper to taste
- Fresh parsley, chopped (for garnish)

Directions:

1. Give the split peas a quick rinse in cold water and reserve.

2. Heat the olive oil in a big pot over medium heat. Add the onion, celery, and carrot, chopped. Cook until the vegetables begin to soften, about 5 minutes.

3. Cook the minced garlic in the pot for a further minute, or until it becomes aromatic.

4. Add the rinsed split peas to the pot with the smoked ham hock. Add the reduced-sodium chicken broth.

5. Include the dried thyme and bay leaf. After bringing the mixture to a boil, lower the heat, cover it, and simmer it for around one and a half hours.

6. Take the ham hock out of the pot after it's soft. Once it cools down a bit, shred the meat, making sure to remove all the bones and fat.

7. Add the shredded ham back to the saucepan. Add salt and pepper to taste when preparing the soup. For ten more minutes, keep simmering.

8. Garnish with fresh parsley and serve hot.

48. Broccoli and Potato Soup

⏰ Time: 55 minutes	🍽 Serving Size: 4 bowls
⚖ Prep Time: 15 minutes	👨‍🍳 Cook Time: 40 minutes

Nutrition Information Per Serving (1 bowl):

Calories: 165, Carbohydrates: 27g, Saturated Fat: 0.5g, Protein: 6g, Fat: 3.5g, Sodium: 70mg, Potassium: 899mg, Fiber: 5g, Sugar: 3g, Vitamin C: 81mg, Calcium: 55mg, Iron: 1.8mg

Ingredients:

- 2 cups broccoli florets
- 1 large potato, peeled and diced
- 1 tablespoon olive oil
- 1 small onion, chopped
- 2 cloves garlic, minced
- 4 cups low-sodium vegetable broth
- Salt and pepper to taste
- Chopped chives for garnish (optional)

Directions:

1. Heat the olive oil in a big pot over medium heat. Add the chopped onion and simmer for about 5 minutes, or until it is tender and transparent.

2. Add the minced garlic and stir until fragrant, about 1 more minute.

3. Stir the broccoli florets and diced potato into the pot with the onion and garlic.

4. Add the veggie broth and heat the blend until it boils. Lower the heat to a simmer and continue cooking for 20 to 25 minutes, or until the potatoes are soft.

5. Puree the soup with an immersion blender until it's creamy after the veggies are tender. In case you don't own an immersion blender, cautiously move the soup into batches and process it in a blender till it becomes smooth.

6. Add salt and pepper to taste when preparing the soup. If desired, top hot dish with chopped chives.

49. Spicy Black Bean Soup

⏰ **Time:** 2 hours	🍽 **Serving Size:** 6 bowls
⏲ **Prep Time:** 15 minutes	👨‍🍳 **Cook Time:** 1 hour 45 min

Nutrition Information Per Serving (1 bowl):

Calories: 210, Carbohydrates: 35g, Saturated Fat: 0.5g, Protein: 13g, Fat: 2g, Sodium: 300mg, Potassium: 800mg, Fiber: 9g, Sugar: 3g, Vitamin C: 5mg, Calcium: 50mg, Iron: 3mg

Ingredients:

- 1 lb dried black beans, rinsed and soaked overnight
- 2 tablespoons olive oil
- 1 large onion, chopped
- 2 bell peppers (any color), diced
- 3 cloves garlic, minced
- 1 jalapeño, seeded and finely chopped (optional)
- 1 teaspoon ground cumin
- 1 teaspoon chili powder
- 1/2 teaspoon dried oregano
- 6 cups low-sodium vegetable broth
- Salt and pepper to taste
- Fresh cilantro, chopped (for garnish)
- Lime wedges (for serving)

Directions:

1. Empty and wash the black beans after soaking.

2. Heat the olive oil in a big pot over medium heat. Add the bell peppers and onion, and sauté for about 5 minutes, or until the veggies are tender.

3. Add the jalapeño, if using, and stir. Cook for a further minute, or until fragrant.

4. Toss in the dried oregano, chili powder, and powdered cumin; toss to coat the vegetables.

5. Add the drained black beans and pour in the vegetable broth. Add pepper and salt for seasoning.

6. After bringing the soup to a boil, lower the heat to a simmer, cover it, and cook the beans for one and a half to two hours, or until they are soft.

7. After the beans are cooked, puree the soup to a partly thicker consistency, leaving some whole beans for texture, using an immersion blender.

8. Present the hot soup with lime wedges and chopped cilantro on the side.

50. Italian Sausage and Tortellini Soup

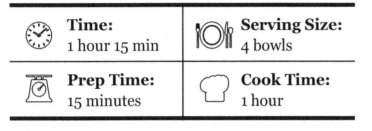

	Time: 1 hour 15 min		Serving Size: 4 bowls
	Prep Time: 15 minutes		Cook Time: 1 hour

Nutrition Information Per Serving (1 bowl):

Calories: 320, Carbohydrates: 38g, Saturated Fat: 3g, Protein: 17g, Fat: 12g, Sodium: 410mg, Potassium: 410mg, Fiber: 4g, Sugar: 5g, Vitamin C: 18mg, Calcium: 150mg, Iron: 2.5mg

Ingredients:

- 1 tablespoon olive oil
- 1/2 pound Italian turkey sausage, casing removed
- 1 small onion, diced
- 2 carrots, peeled and diced
- 2 stalks celery, diced
- 3 cloves garlic, minced
- 1 teaspoon dried oregano
- 1 teaspoon dried basil
- 4 cups low-sodium chicken broth
- 1 (14.5-ounce) can diced tomatoes, no salt added
- 1 cup fresh spinach, chopped
- 9 ounces refrigerated cheese tortellini
- Salt and pepper to taste
- Grated Parmesan cheese for serving (optional)

Directions:

1. Heat the olive oil in a large pot over medium heat. Add the Italian turkey sausage and cook, breaking it up with a spoon, until browned, about 5 minutes.

2. Add the diced onion, carrots, and celery to the pot and cook until the vegetables are softened, about 10 minutes.

3. Stir in the minced garlic, dried oregano, and dried basil, and cook for another 2 minutes.

4. Pour in the chicken broth and add the can of diced tomatoes with their juice. Bring the soup to a boil, then reduce the heat and let it simmer for 30 minutes.

5. Add the chopped spinach and cheese tortellini to the pot. Simmer for another 10 minutes, or until the tortellini is cooked through.

6. Season with salt and pepper to taste. Serve hot, sprinkled with grated Parmesan cheese if desired.

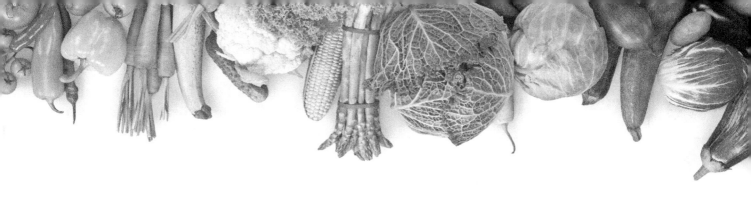

CHAPTER 7: MEAT

51. Beef Stir Fry with Broccoli and Bell Peppers

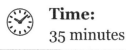 **Time:** 35 minutes	**Serving Size:** 4
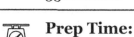 **Prep Time:** 15 minutes	**Cook Time:** 20 minutes

Nutrition Information Per Serving (1 serving unit):

Calories: 250, Carbohydrates: 12g, Saturated Fat: 2g, Protein: 28g, Fat: 10g, Sodium: 300mg, Potassium: 800mg, Fiber: 3g, Sugar: 5g, Vitamin C: 130mg, Calcium: 50mg, Iron: 3mg

Ingredients:

- 1 pound lean beef, thinly sliced
- 2 cups broccoli florets
- 1 red bell pepper, sliced
- 1 yellow bell pepper, sliced
- 1 tablespoon low-sodium soy sauce
- 2 teaspoons cornstarch
- 1 tablespoon olive oil
- 1 teaspoon ginger, minced
- 2 cloves garlic, minced
- 1/2 cup low-sodium beef broth
- Salt and pepper to taste

Directions:

1. In a small bowl, whisk together the low-sodium soy sauce, cornstarch, and low-sodium beef broth until the cornstarch is fully dissolved. Set aside.

2. Season the sliced beef with a pinch of salt and pepper.

3. Heat the olive oil in a large skillet or wok over medium-high heat.

4. Add the minced garlic and ginger to the skillet and sauté for about 30 seconds or until fragrant.

5. Add the beef to the skillet and stir-fry for about 3-4 minutes or until it is browned and cooked through.

6. Remove the beef from the skillet and set aside on a plate.

7. In the same skillet, add the broccoli and bell pepper slices. Stir-fry for about 5 minutes or until the vegetables are tender but still crisp.

8. Return the beef to the skillet with the vegetables.

9. Stir in the soy sauce mixture, and continue to cook for another 2 minutes or until the sauce has thickened and everything is well coated.

10. Taste and adjust seasoning if necessary.

11. Serve hot, and enjoy your flavorful, pancreatitis-friendly beef stir fry!

52. Chicken Cacciatore

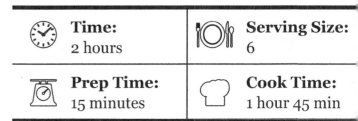 **Time:** 1 hour 10 min	**Serving Size:** 4
Prep Time: 20 minutes	**Cook Time:** 50 minutes

Nutrition Information Per Serving (1 serving unit):

Calories: 310, Carbohydrates: 15g, Saturated Fat: 1g, Protein: 35g, Fat: 12g, Sodium: 410mg, Potassium: 650mg, Fiber: 3g, Sugar: 7g, Vitamin C: 25mg, Calcium: 40mg, Iron: 2mg

Ingredients:

- 4 boneless, skinless chicken breasts
- 1 tablespoon olive oil
- 1 small onion, diced
- 2 cloves garlic, minced
- 1 bell pepper, sliced
- 1 (14.5-ounce) can no-salt-added diced tomatoes
- 1/2 cup low-sodium chicken broth
- 1 teaspoon dried oregano
- 1 teaspoon dried basil
- 1/2 teaspoon salt
- 1/4 teaspoon black pepper
- 1/4 cup chopped fresh parsley
- 1/2 cup sliced mushrooms

Directions:

1. Preheat your oven to 350°F.
2. In a large ovenproof skillet, heat the olive oil over medium-high heat. Add the chicken breasts and cook until browned on both sides, about 3-4 minutes per side. Remove chicken and set aside.
3. In the same skillet, add the onion, garlic, and bell pepper, and sauté until the vegetables are softened, about 5 minutes.
4. Stir in the diced tomatoes, chicken broth, oregano, basil, salt, and black pepper, and bring to a simmer.
5. Return the chicken to the skillet and sprinkle the mushrooms over the top.
6. Cover the skillet with a lid or aluminum foil and bake in the preheated oven for 40-45 minutes, or until the chicken is cooked through and reaches an internal temperature of 165°F.
7. Garnish with fresh parsley before serving.

53. Roast Beef with Root Vegetables

Time: 2 hours	**Serving Size:** 6
Prep Time: 15 minutes	**Cook Time:** 1 hour 45 min

Nutrition Information Per Serving (1 serving unit):

Calories: 330, Carbohydrates: 18g, Saturated Fat: 3g, Protein: 45g, Fat: 9g, Sodium: 120mg, Potassium: 980mg, Fiber: 3g, Sugar: 5g, Vitamin C: 19mg, Calcium: 50mg, Iron: 4mg

Ingredients:

- 2 pounds beef eye round roast
- 1 tablespoon olive oil
- 1 teaspoon garlic powder
- 1 teaspoon dried rosemary
- 1/2 teaspoon salt
- 1/2 teaspoon ground black pepper
- 3 medium carrots, peeled and cut into 2-inch pieces
- 2 medium parsnips, peeled and cut into 2-inch pieces
- 1 medium turnip, peeled and cut into wedges
- 1/2 pound small red potatoes, quartered
- 1/2 cup low-sodium beef broth

Directions:

1. Preheat your oven to 375°F.

2. Rub the beef roast with olive oil, and then evenly sprinkle garlic powder, dried rosemary, salt, and black pepper over the surface.

3. Place the seasoned beef in a roasting pan.

4. In a large bowl, toss the carrots, parsnips, turnip, and red potatoes with any remaining olive oil and additional salt and pepper if desired.

5. Arrange the vegetables around the beef in the roasting pan.

6. Pour the beef broth over the vegetables, which will help to steam them while roasting and add flavor.

7. Roast in the preheated oven for about 1 hour and 45 minutes, or until the beef reaches an internal temperature of 145°F for medium-rare.

8. Remove from the oven and let the roast beef rest for at least 10 minutes before slicing. This allows the juices to redistribute.

9. Serve the beef sliced with the roasted root vegetables on the side.

54. Meatloaf with Turkey and Quinoa

⏰	**Time:** 1 hour 30 min	🍽️	**Serving Size:** 6
⚖️	**Prep Time:** 20 minutes	👨‍🍳	**Cook Time:** 1 hour 10 min

Nutrition Information Per Serving (1 serving unit):

Calories: 220, Carbohydrates: 15g, Saturated Fat: 1.5g, Protein: 28g, Fat: 7g, Sodium: 240mg, Potassium: 370mg, Fiber: 2g, Sugar: 3g, Vitamin C: 1.2mg, Calcium: 30mg, Iron: 2.4mg

Ingredients:

- 1 pound ground turkey breast
- 1 cup cooked quinoa
- 1/2 cup finely chopped onion
- 1/2 cup grated carrot
- 1/2 cup finely chopped bell pepper
- 2 cloves garlic, minced
- 1 egg, beaten
- 2 tablespoons tomato paste
- 1 tablespoon Worcestershire sauce
- 1 teaspoon dried thyme
- 1 teaspoon dried oregano
- 1/2 teaspoon salt
- 1/4 teaspoon ground black pepper
- 1/4 cup low-sodium chicken broth

Directions:

1. Preheat your oven to 350°F.

2. In a large bowl, combine the ground turkey breast, cooked quinoa, finely chopped onion, grated carrot, finely chopped bell pepper, and minced garlic.

3. In a separate small bowl, whisk together the beaten egg, tomato paste, Worcestershire sauce, dried thyme, dried oregano, salt, and ground black pepper.

4. Pour the egg mixture into the turkey mixture and mix until just combined.

5. Gradually mix in the low-sodium chicken broth to keep the mixture moist.

6. Transfer the mixture into a loaf pan that has been lightly greased or lined with parchment paper.

7. Bake in the preheated oven for 70 minutes or until the meatloaf is cooked through and reaches an internal temperature of 165°F.

8. Let the meatloaf rest for 10 minutes before slicing and serving.

55. Lemon Herb Roasted Chicken

 Time: 1 hour 35 min	 Serving Size: 4
 Prep Time: 15 minutes	 Cook Time: 1 hour 20 min

Nutrition Information Per Serving (1 serving unit):

Calories: 275, Carbohydrates: 5g, Saturated Fat: 1g, Protein: 35g, Fat: 13g, Sodium: 180mg, Potassium: 370mg, Fiber: 1g, Sugar: 1g, Vitamin C: 6mg, Calcium: 30mg, Iron: 2mg

Ingredients:

- 4 boneless, skinless chicken breasts
- 2 tablespoons olive oil
- 4 garlic cloves, minced
- 1 teaspoon dried thyme
- 1 lemon, sliced
- 1 teaspoon dried rosemary
- 1/2 teaspoon salt
- 1/4 teaspoon black pepper
- 1/2 cup low-sodium chicken broth

Directions:

1. Preheat your oven to 375°F.
2. In a bowl, mix together olive oil, minced garlic, thyme, rosemary, salt, and black pepper to create the herb mixture.
3. Place the chicken breasts in a baking dish and rub them evenly with the herb mixture.
4. Arrange the lemon slices over and around the chicken in the dish.
5. Pour the chicken broth into the base of the dish, being careful not to wash the herb mixture off the chicken.
6. Roast in the preheated oven for approximately 70-80 minutes, or until the chicken is cooked through and reaches an internal temperature of 165°F.
7. Let the chicken rest for 5 minutes before serving to allow the juices to redistribute.

56. Pork Chops with Peach Salsa

 Time: 25 minutes	 Serving Size: 4 chops
 Prep Time: 10 minutes	 Cook Time: 15 minutes

Nutrition Information Per Serving (1 chop):

Calories: 220, Carbohydrates: 14g, Saturated Fat: 1g, Protein: 25g, Fat: 7g, Sodium: 320mg, Potassium: 570mg, Fiber: 2g, Sugar: 11g, Vitamin C: 10mg, Calcium: 20mg, Iron: 1mg

Ingredients:

- 4 boneless pork chops, 1/2 inch thick
- 2 teaspoons olive oil
- Salt and pepper to taste
- 2 peaches, pitted and diced
- 1/4 cup red onion, finely chopped
- 1/4 cup fresh cilantro, chopped
- 1 tablespoon fresh lime juice
- 1 teaspoon honey
- 1/4 teaspoon chili flakes (optional)

Directions:

1. Preheat the grill to medium-high heat or an indoor grill pan to 375°F.
2. Season both sides of the pork chops with salt and pepper.
3. Brush the grill with olive oil to prevent sticking and place the pork chops on the grill.
4. Grill the pork chops for about 6-7 minutes on each side, or until the internal temperature reaches 145°F.

5. While the pork chops are grilling, prepare the peach salsa by combining the diced peaches, red onion, cilantro, lime juice, honey, and chili flakes (if using) in a bowl. Mix well and set aside.

6. Once the pork chops are cooked, remove them from the grill and let them rest for a few minutes.

7. Serve the pork chops topped with the fresh peach salsa.

57. Beef and Mushroom Skillet

⏱ **Time:** 1 hour	🍽 **Serving Size:** 4
⚖ **Prep Time:** 15 minutes	🍞 **Cook Time:** 45 minutes

Nutrition Information Per Serving (1 serving unit):

Calories: 310, Carbohydrates: 9g, Saturated Fat: 2g, Protein: 35g, Fat: 15g, Sodium: 320mg, Potassium: 650mg, Fiber: 2g, Sugar: 4g, Vitamin C: 2mg, Calcium: 20mg, Iron: 3mg

Ingredients:

- 1 pound lean beef, cut into strips
- 2 cups sliced mushrooms
- 1 medium onion, diced
- 2 cloves garlic, minced
- 1 tablespoon olive oil
- 1/2 cup low-sodium beef broth
- 1 tablespoon Worcestershire sauce
- 1 teaspoon dried thyme
- 1/2 teaspoon salt
- 1/4 teaspoon black pepper
- 2 tablespoons chopped fresh parsley (for garnish)

Directions:

1. Heat olive oil in a large skillet over medium-high heat.

2. Add the beef strips to the skillet and cook until browned on all sides, about 5 minutes. Remove the beef from the skillet and set aside.

3. In the same skillet, add the diced onion and minced garlic, and sauté until the onion is translucent, about 3 minutes.

4. Add the sliced mushrooms to the skillet and cook until they are soft and browned, about 5 minutes.

5. Return the beef to the skillet with the mushrooms and onions.

6. Pour in the low-sodium beef broth and Worcestershire sauce, and then season with dried thyme, salt, and black pepper.

7. Stir well to combine and bring to a simmer. Reduce heat to low and cook for 30 minutes, stirring occasionally.

8. Garnish with chopped fresh parsley before serving.

58. Chicken Fajitas with Whole Wheat Tortillas

⏱ **Time:** 45 minutes	🍽 **Serving Size:** 4 fajitas
⚖ **Prep Time:** 15 minutes	🍞 **Cook Time:** 30 minutes

Nutrition Information Per Serving (1 fajita):

Calories: 320, Carbohydrates: 34g, Saturated Fat: 2g, Protein: 27g, Fat: 9g, Sodium: 490mg, Potassium: 495mg, Fiber: 5g, Sugar: 3g, Vitamin C: 60mg, Calcium: 80mg, Iron: 2mg

Ingredients:

- 1 pound boneless, skinless chicken breasts, thinly sliced
- 1 tablespoon olive oil
- 1 red bell pepper, sliced
- 1 green bell pepper, sliced
- 1 yellow onion, sliced
- 2 cloves garlic, minced
- 1 teaspoon ground cumin
- 1 teaspoon paprika
- 1/2 teaspoon dried oregano
- 1/4 teaspoon chili powder (optional)
- 1/4 teaspoon salt
- 1/4 teaspoon black pepper
- 8 whole wheat tortillas
- Fresh cilantro, for garnish
- Lime wedges, for serving

Directions:

1. In a large bowl, combine the chicken slices with cumin, paprika, oregano, chili powder (if using), salt, and black pepper.

2. Heat olive oil in a large skillet over medium-high heat. Add the seasoned chicken to the skillet and cook for about 5-6 minutes until browned and cooked through. Remove chicken from the skillet and set aside.

3. In the same skillet, add a bit more olive oil if needed, and sauté the bell peppers, onion, and garlic for about 4-5 minutes until they are soft and slightly caramelized.

4. Return the chicken to the skillet with the vegetables and stir to combine. Cook for an additional 2-3 minutes.

5. Warm the whole wheat tortillas in a separate pan or in the microwave.

6. Spoon the chicken and vegetable mixture into the center of each tortilla. Garnish with fresh cilantro.

7. Serve the fajitas with lime wedges on the side.

59. Turkey Burger with Avocado

🕐 **Time:** 40 minutes	🍽 **Serving Size:** 4 burger
⚖ **Prep Time:** 10 minutes	👨‍🍳 **Cook Time:** 30 minutes

Nutrition Information Per Serving (1 burger):

Calories: 260, Carbohydrates: 22g, Saturated Fat: 2g, Protein: 26g, Fat: 9g, Sodium: 430mg, Potassium: 670mg, Fiber: 6g, Sugar: 3g, Vitamin C: 8mg, Calcium: 50mg, Iron: 2mg

Ingredients:

- 1 pound ground turkey breast
- 1 ripe avocado, sliced
- 4 whole wheat hamburger buns
- 1 tablespoon olive oil
- 1 teaspoon garlic powder
- 1 teaspoon onion powder
- 1/2 teaspoon paprika
- Salt and pepper to taste
- Lettuce leaves
- 1 tomato, sliced
- 1 red onion, thinly sliced

Directions:

1. Preheat your grill to medium-high heat, around 375°F.

2. In a bowl, mix the ground turkey with garlic powder, onion powder, paprika, salt, and pepper.

3. Form the mixture into 4 equal-sized patties.

4. Brush each patty lightly with olive oil to prevent sticking to the grill.

5. Place the turkey patties on the grill and cook for about 6-7 minutes on each side or until the internal temperature reaches 165°F.

6. During the last few minutes of cooking, place the whole wheat buns, cut side down, on the grill to toast lightly.

7. To assemble the burgers, place a lettuce leaf on the bottom half of each bun, followed by a cooked turkey patty.

8. Top each patty with sliced avocado, tomato, and red onion.

9. Cover with the top half of the bun and serve immediately.

60. Slow Cooker Pulled Pork

⏰ **Time:** 6 hours	🍽 **Serving Size:** 6
⚖ **Prep Time:** 15 minutes	👨‍🍳 **Cook Time:** 7 hours 45 min

Nutrition Information Per Serving (1 serving):

Calories: 210, Carbohydrates: 5g, Saturated Fat: 1g, Protein: 30g, Fat: 8g, Sodium: 290mg, Potassium: 500mg, Fiber: 1g, Sugar: 2g, Vitamin C: 1mg, Calcium: 20mg, Iron: 1.5mg

Ingredients:

- 2 pounds pork tenderloin
- 1 cup low-sodium chicken broth
- 1 medium onion, thinly sliced
- 3 cloves garlic, minced
- 1 tablespoon honey
- 1 tablespoon apple cider vinegar
- 1 teaspoon smoked paprika
- 1 teaspoon mustard powder
- 1/2 teaspoon ground cumin
- 1/2 teaspoon black pepper
- 1/4 teaspoon salt
- 2 tablespoons chopped fresh parsley (for garnish)

Directions:

1. Place the pork tenderloin in the slow cooker.

2. In a small bowl, mix together the honey, apple cider vinegar, smoked paprika, mustard powder, ground cumin, black pepper, and salt to create a marinade.

3. Pour the marinade over the pork in the slow cooker.

4. Add the thinly sliced onion and minced garlic to the slow cooker, spreading them around the pork.

5. Pour the low-sodium chicken broth into the slow cooker.

6. Cover and cook on low for 7 to 8 hours, or until the pork is tender and shreds easily with a fork.

7. Remove the pork from the slow cooker and shred it using two forks.

8. If desired, skim the fat from the cooking juices and pour some of the juices over the shredded pork to keep it moist.

9. Garnish with chopped fresh parsley before serving.

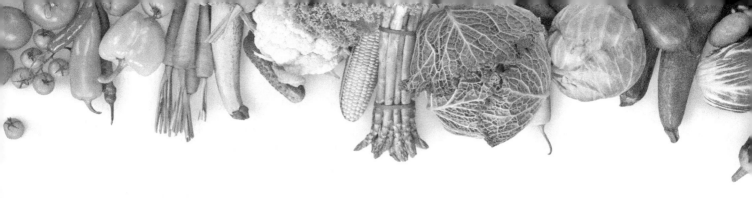

CHAPTER 8: FISH AND SEAFOOD

61. Baked Salmon with Dill and Lemon

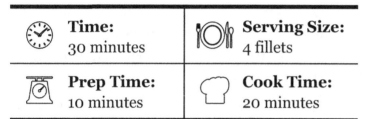 Time: 30 minutes	Serving Size: 4 fillets
Prep Time: 10 minutes	Cook Time: 20 minutes

Nutrition Information Per Serving (1 fillet):

Calories: 295, Carbohydrates: 0g, Saturated Fat: 3g, Protein: 23g, Fat: 22g, Sodium: 50mg, Potassium: 555mg, Fiber: 0g, Sugar: 0g, Vitamin C: 0.1mg, Calcium: 14mg, Iron: 0.8mg

Ingredients:

- 4 salmon fillets (4 ounces each)
- 2 tablespoons fresh dill, chopped
- 1 lemon, thinly sliced
- 1 tablespoon olive oil
- Salt and pepper to taste

Directions:

1. Preheat your oven to 375°F.
2. Line a baking sheet with parchment paper for easy cleanup.
3. Place the salmon fillets on the prepared baking sheet.
4. Brush each fillet with olive oil and season with salt and pepper.
5. Sprinkle chopped dill evenly over the salmon fillets.
6. Arrange lemon slices on top of the seasoned fillets.
7. Bake in the preheated oven for 15-20 minutes, or until the salmon flakes easily with a fork.
8. Serve hot, garnished with additional fresh dill if desired.

62. Shrimp and Asparagus Stir Fry

Time: 30 minutes	Serving Size: 4 plates
Prep Time: 10 minutes	Cook Time: 20 minutes

Nutrition Information Per Serving (1 plate):

Calories: 180, Carbohydrates: 7g, Saturated Fat: 1g, Protein: 24g, Fat: 7g, Sodium: 330mg, Potassium: 300mg, Fiber: 3g, Sugar: 2g, Vitamin C: 12mg, Calcium: 100mg, Iron: 2.5mg

Ingredients:

- 1 pound large shrimp, peeled and deveined
- 1 bunch asparagus, trimmed and cut into 2-inch pieces
- 1 tablespoon olive oil
- 2 cloves garlic, minced
- 1 teaspoon ginger, grated
- 2 tablespoons low-sodium soy sauce
- 1 tablespoon oyster sauce
- 1 teaspoon sesame oil
- 1/4 cup low-sodium chicken broth
- Salt and pepper to taste
- 1 tablespoon sesame seeds (for garnish)
- 1 green onion, thinly sliced (for garnish)

Directions:

1. Heat olive oil in a large skillet or wok over medium-high heat.

2. Add the minced garlic and grated ginger, sautéing for about 30 seconds until fragrant.

3. Toss in the asparagus and stir-fry for 3-4 minutes until they're tender-crisp.

4. Push the asparagus to the side of the skillet and add the shrimp, cooking for about 2 minutes on each side or until they turn pink.

5. In a small bowl, whisk together the low-sodium soy sauce, oyster sauce, sesame oil, and chicken broth.

6. Pour the sauce mixture over the shrimp and asparagus, tossing everything together to coat well and heat through for another 2 minutes.

7. Season with salt and pepper to taste.

8. Garnish with sesame seeds and sliced green onion before serving.

63. Grilled Tilapia with Mango Salsa

⏰ **Time:** 25 minutes	🍽 **Serving Size:** 4 fillets
⚖ **Prep Time:** 15 minutes	👨‍🍳 **Cook Time:** 10 minutes

Nutrition Information Per Serving (1 fillet):

Calories: 210, Carbohydrates: 9g, Saturated Fat: 1.5g, Protein: 35g, Fat: 4g, Sodium: 85mg, Potassium: 830mg, Fiber: 1g, Sugar: 7g, Vitamin C: 38mg, Calcium: 20mg, Iron: 1.4mg

Ingredients:

- 4 tilapia fillets (6 ounces each)
- 1 ripe mango, peeled, pitted, and diced
- 1/2 red bell pepper, diced
- 1/4 cup red onion, finely chopped
- 1 small jalapeño, seeded and minced (optional)
- 1/4 cup fresh cilantro, chopped
- Juice of 1 lime
- 1 tablespoon olive oil
- Salt and pepper to taste

Directions:

1. Preheat your grill to medium-high heat.

2. In a medium bowl, combine mango, red bell pepper, red onion, jalapeño (if using), cilantro, and lime juice. Season with salt to taste and set aside to let the flavors meld, creating the mango salsa.

3. Brush both sides of the tilapia fillets with olive oil and season with salt and pepper.

4. Place tilapia on the grill and cook for about 4-5 minutes on each side, or until the fish flakes easily with a fork.

5. Remove the tilapia from the grill and let it rest for a minute.

6. Serve the grilled tilapia topped with the fresh mango salsa.

64. Sea Bass with Mediterranean Vegetables

⏰ Time: 40 minutes	🍽 Serving Size: 4
⚖ Prep Time: 15 minutes	👨‍🍳 Cook Time: 25 minutes

Nutrition Information Per Serving (1 serving):

Calories: 280, Carbohydrates: 10g, Saturated Fat: 1g, Protein: 28g, Fat: 16g, Sodium: 120mg, Potassium: 650mg, Fiber: 3g, Sugar: 4g, Vitamin C: 25mg, Calcium: 40mg, Iron: 1.2mg

Ingredients:

- 4 sea bass fillets (6 ounces each)
- 2 zucchinis, sliced into half-moons
- 1 yellow bell pepper, diced
- 1 cup cherry tomatoes, halved
- 1/4 cup Kalamata olives, pitted and halved
- 2 tablespoons capers, rinsed
- 1 tablespoon olive oil
- 2 cloves garlic, minced
- Juice of 1 lemon
- 1 teaspoon dried oregano
- Salt and pepper to taste
- Fresh parsley, chopped (for garnish)

Directions:

1. Preheat your oven to 400°F.
2. In a large bowl, combine zucchini, yellow bell pepper, cherry tomatoes, Kalamata olives, capers, and minced garlic.
3. Drizzle with olive oil and lemon juice, then sprinkle with oregano, salt, and pepper. Toss to coat the vegetables evenly.
4. Spread the vegetables in a single layer on a baking sheet and roast for 10 minutes.
5. Remove the baking sheet from the oven and place the sea bass fillets among the vegetables.
6. Return the baking sheet to the oven and roast for an additional 12-15 minutes, or until the sea bass is cooked through and flakes easily with a fork.
7. Serve the sea bass hot, garnished with fresh parsley.

65. Tuna Salad with Greek Yogurt

⏰ Time: 15 minutes	🍽 Serving Size: 4
⚖ Prep Time: 10 minutes	👨‍🍳 Cook Time: 5 minutes

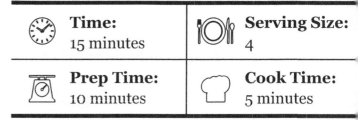

Nutrition Information Per Serving (1 serving unit):

Calories: 150, Carbohydrates: 6g, Saturated Fat: 0.5g, Protein: 22g, Fat: 4g, Sodium: 210mg, Potassium: 240mg, Fiber: 1g, Sugar: 3g, Vitamin C: 5mg, Calcium: 60mg, Iron: 1.2mg

Ingredients:

- 2 cans (5 ounces each) no-salt-added tuna in water, drained
- 1/2 cup nonfat Greek yogurt
- 1/4 cup celery, finely chopped
- 1/4 cup red onion, finely chopped
- 1 tablespoon fresh lemon juice
- 1 tablespoon fresh dill, chopped
- 1/4 teaspoon garlic powder
- Salt and pepper to taste
- Lettuce leaves or whole-grain bread for serving

Directions:

1. In a medium-sized mixing bowl, flake the drained tuna with a fork.

2. Add the nonfat Greek yogurt to the tuna and mix until well combined.

3. Stir in the finely chopped celery and red onion, ensuring the ingredients are evenly distributed throughout the tuna mixture.

4. Season the mixture with fresh lemon juice, chopped dill, and garlic powder. Mix well.

5. Taste and adjust the seasoning with salt and pepper as desired.

6. Serve the tuna salad on a bed of lettuce leaves for a low-carbohydrate option or spread it on whole-grain bread for a hearty sandwich.

66. Mussels in Tomato and Garlic Broth

⏱	**Time:** 35 minutes	🍽	**Serving Size:** 4
⚖	**Prep Time:** 15 minutes	👨‍🍳	**Cook Time:** 20 minutes

Nutrition Information Per Serving (1 serving):

Calories: 180, Carbohydrates: 10g, Saturated Fat: 1g, Protein: 18g, Fat: 6g, Sodium: 340mg, Potassium: 400mg, Fiber: 1g, Sugar: 4g, Vitamin C: 15mg, Calcium: 40mg, Iron: 5mg

Ingredients:

- 2 pounds fresh mussels, cleaned and debearded
- 1 tablespoon olive oil
- 3 cloves garlic, minced
- 1 small onion, diced
- 1 can (14 ounces) no-salt-added diced tomatoes
- 1 cup low-sodium vegetable broth
- 1/4 cup fresh parsley, chopped
- 1 teaspoon dried thyme
- 1/2 teaspoon red pepper flakes (optional)
- Salt and pepper to taste
- Lemon wedges for serving

Directions:

1. In a large pot, heat the olive oil over medium heat. Add the garlic and onion, and sauté until the onion is translucent, about 3 minutes.

2. Stir in the diced tomatoes, vegetable broth, parsley, thyme, and red pepper flakes if using. Season with salt and pepper to taste.

3. Bring the mixture to a simmer and let it cook for 10 minutes to allow the flavors to meld.

4. Add the cleaned mussels to the pot, cover with a lid, and cook for about 5-7 minutes, or until the mussels have opened. Discard any mussels that do not open.

5. Serve the mussels in bowls with plenty of the tomato and garlic broth. Garnish with additional chopped parsley and lemon wedges on the side.

67. Crab Cakes with Remoulade Sauce

⏰ **Time:** 45 minutes	🍽 **Serving Size:** 4 cakes
⚖ **Prep Time:** 20 minutes	👨‍🍳 **Cook Time:** 25 minutes

Nutrition Information Per Serving (1 cake):

Calories: 210, Carbohydrates: 12g, Saturated Fat: 1g, Protein: 16g, Fat: 10g, Sodium: 380mg, Potassium: 370mg, Fiber: 1g, Sugar: 2g, Vitamin C: 4mg, Calcium: 85mg, Iron: 0.7mg

Ingredients:

- 1 pound lump crabmeat, carefully picked over for shells
- 1/4 cup whole wheat breadcrumbs
- 1/4 cup finely chopped green onions
- 1/4 cup finely chopped red bell pepper
- 1 egg white
- 1 tablespoon low-fat mayonnaise
- 1 teaspoon Dijon mustard
- 1 teaspoon Worcestershire sauce
- 1/2 teaspoon Old Bay seasoning
- 1/4 teaspoon ground black pepper
- 2 tablespoons olive oil for cooking

For the Remoulade Sauce:

- 1/2 cup fat-free mayonnaise
- 1 tablespoon capers, rinsed and chopped
- 1 tablespoon Dijon mustard
- 1 tablespoon minced fresh parsley
- 1 teaspoon lemon juice
- 1/4 teaspoon paprika
- 1/4 teaspoon garlic powder

Directions:

1. In a large bowl, combine crabmeat, breadcrumbs, green onions, and red bell pepper.

2. In a separate small bowl, whisk together egg white, low-fat mayonnaise, Dijon mustard, Worcestershire sauce, Old Bay seasoning, and black pepper.

3. Fold the egg mixture into the crab mixture until well combined, being careful not to overmix.

4. Form the mixture into 8 equal-sized patties.

5. Heat olive oil in a large non-stick skillet over medium heat.

6. Cook crab cakes in batches for about 3 to 5 minutes on each side, or until golden brown and heated through.

7. For the remoulade sauce, mix together fat-free mayonnaise, capers, Dijon mustard, parsley, lemon juice, paprika, and garlic powder in a small bowl.

8. Serve crab cakes with a dollop of remoulade sauce on top or on the side for dipping.

68. Clam Chowder with Corn and Potatoes

⏰ **Time:** 55 minutes	🍽 **Serving Size:** 4
⚖ **Prep Time:** 15 minutes	👨‍🍳 **Cook Time:** 40 minutes

Nutrition Information Per Serving (1 serving):

Calories: 250, Carbohydrates: 35g, Saturated Fat: 1g, Protein: 14g, Fat: 5g, Sodium: 480mg, Potassium: 720mg, Fiber: 4g, Sugar: 5g, Vitamin C: 12mg, Calcium: 50mg, Iron: 2mg

Ingredients:

- 2 cans (6.5 ounces each) chopped clams in juice
- 2 cups diced potatoes
- 1 cup corn kernels, fresh or frozen
- 1 cup diced celery
- 1 cup diced onion
- 2 cloves garlic, minced
- 2 cups low-fat milk
- 1 cup low-sodium vegetable broth
- 2 tablespoons cornstarch
- 1 tablespoon olive oil
- 1/2 teaspoon dried thyme
- Salt and pepper to taste
- Fresh parsley, chopped (for garnish)

Directions:

1. Drain the clams, reserving the juice. Set aside.

2. In a large pot, heat the olive oil over medium heat. Add the onion, celery, and garlic, and sauté until the vegetables are tender, about 5 minutes.

3. Add the potatoes, corn, thyme, reserved clam juice, and vegetable broth to the pot. Bring to a boil, then reduce heat and simmer until the potatoes are tender, about 20 minutes.

4. In a small bowl, whisk together the cornstarch with 1/4 cup of water to create a slurry. Stir the slurry into the chowder to thicken it.

5. Add the milk and clams to the pot. Cook until heated through, but do not boil, for about 5 minutes.

6. Season with salt and pepper to taste. Serve hot, garnished with fresh parsley.

69. Grilled Sardines with Lemon and Herbs

⏰ **Time:** 30 minutes	🍽 **Serving Size:** 4 sardines
⚖ **Prep Time:** 10 minutes	👨‍🍳 **Cook Time:** 20 minutes

Nutrition Information Per Serving (1 sardine):

Calories: 190, Carbohydrates: 1g, Saturated Fat: 1g, Protein: 25g, Fat: 10g, Sodium: 200mg, Potassium: 450mg, Fiber: 0g, Sugar: 0g, Vitamin C: 20mg, Calcium: 300mg, Iron: 2.5mg

Ingredients:

- 1 pound fresh sardines, cleaned and gutted
- 2 tablespoons fresh lemon juice
- 2 cloves garlic, minced
- 1 tablespoon chopped fresh parsley
- 1 tablespoon chopped fresh basil
- 1 teaspoon chopped fresh oregano
- 2 tablespoons olive oil
- 1/2 teaspoon sea salt
- 1/4 teaspoon black pepper
- Lemon wedges for garnish

Directions:

1. Preheat your grill to medium-high heat, around 375°F.

2. In a small bowl, mix together the lemon juice, minced garlic, parsley, basil, oregano, and olive oil to create a marinade.

3. Lay the sardines in a shallow dish and pour the marinade over them, ensuring they are well coated. Sprinkle with sea salt and black pepper.

4. Let the sardines marinate for 10 minutes.

5. Place the sardines on the grill and cook for about 10 minutes on each side, or until the skin is crispy and the fish is cooked through.

6. Serve the grilled sardines with additional lemon wedges for squeezing over the top.

70. Fish Tacos with Cabbage Slaw

⏰ **Time:** 35 minutes	🍽 **Serving Size:** 4 tacos
⚖ **Prep Time:** 15 minutes	👨‍🍳 **Cook Time:** 20 minutes

Nutrition Information Per Serving (1 taco):

Calories: 310, Carbohydrates: 34g, Saturated Fat: 1g, Protein: 26g, Fat: 9g, Sodium: 210mg, Potassium: 558mg, Fiber: 5g, Sugar: 4g, Vitamin C: 25mg, Calcium: 85mg, Iron: 2mg

Ingredients:

- 1 pound white fish fillets (like tilapia, cod, or mahi-mahi)
- 8 small corn tortillas
- 2 cups shredded cabbage
- 1 medium carrot, shredded
- 1/4 cup chopped fresh cilantro
- 1 lime, juiced
- 1 tablespoon olive oil
- 1 teaspoon ground cumin
- 1/2 teaspoon paprika
- 1/2 teaspoon garlic powder
- Salt and pepper to taste
- Lime wedges for serving

Directions:

1. Preheat the oven to 375°F. Line a baking sheet with parchment paper.

2. In a small bowl, combine the cumin, paprika, garlic powder, salt, and pepper. Sprinkle the seasoning mix over both sides of the fish fillets.

3. Place the seasoned fish on the prepared baking sheet and drizzle with olive oil. Bake for 15-20 minutes or until the fish is flaky and cooked through.

4. While the fish is baking, in a medium bowl, toss together the shredded cabbage, carrot, cilantro, and lime juice. Season with salt and pepper to taste. This will be your cabbage slaw.

5. Warm the corn tortillas in the oven for the last 5 minutes of the fish's cook time or until they are soft and pliable.

6. Once the fish is done, use a fork to flake it into bite-sized pieces.

7. Assemble the tacos by placing an equal amount of fish and cabbage slaw on each tortilla. Serve with lime wedges on the side.

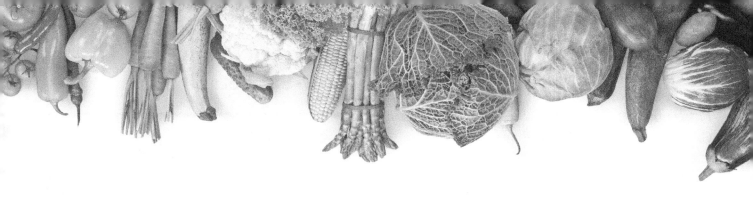

CHAPTER 9: SALADS AND SIDE DISHES

71. Arugula and Beet Salad with Walnuts

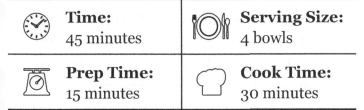

⏰ Time: 45 minutes	🍽 Serving Size: 4 bowls
⏲ Prep Time: 15 minutes	👨‍🍳 Cook Time: 30 minutes

Nutrition Information Per Serving (1 bowl):

Calories: 150, Carbohydrates: 17g, Saturated Fat: 1g, Protein: 4g, Fat: 8g, Sodium: 130mg, Potassium: 369mg, Fiber: 4g, Sugar: 9g, Vitamin C: 10mg, Calcium: 60mg, Iron: 1.5mg

Ingredients:

- 4 medium beets, trimmed and scrubbed
- 4 cups arugula, washed and dried
- 1/4 cup walnuts, chopped
- 1 small red onion, thinly sliced
- 2 tablespoons balsamic vinegar
- 1 tablespoon extra-virgin olive oil
- 1/2 teaspoon Dijon mustard
- Salt and pepper to taste

Directions:

1. Set oven temperature to 400°F.

2. Put the beets on a baking sheet and cover them with aluminum foil. Bake in the preheated oven for approximately half an hour, or until the biggest beets are readily cut with a knife.

3. After roasting, let the beets cool before peeling and chopping them into small pieces.

4. Diced beets, walnuts, red onion, and arugula should all be combined in a big bowl.

5. To make the dressing, combine the olive oil, Dijon mustard, balsamic vinegar, salt, and pepper in a small bowl.

6. After drizzling the salad with the dressing, gently toss to coat.

7. To accentuate the tastes, serve the salad right away or let it cool in the refrigerator for half an hour before serving.

72. Quinoa Salad with Black Beans and Corn

⏰ Time: 30 minutes	🍽 Serving Size: 4 bowls
⏲ Prep Time: 10 minutes	👨‍🍳 Cook Time: 20 minutes

Nutrition Information Per Serving (1 bowl):

Calories: 220, Carbohydrates: 40g, Saturated Fat: 0.5g, Protein: 9g, Fat: 3g, Sodium: 15mg, Potassium: 332mg, Fiber: 8g, Sugar: 2g, Vitamin C: 1.2mg, Calcium: 30mg, Iron: 2.5mg

Ingredients:

- 1 cup quinoa, rinsed
- 2 cups water
- 1 cup canned black beans, drained and rinsed
- 1 cup corn kernels, fresh or frozen
- 1 red bell pepper, diced
- 1/4 cup fresh cilantro, chopped
- 1 lime, juiced
- 1 tablespoon extra-virgin olive oil
- 1/2 teaspoon ground cumin
- Salt and pepper to taste

Directions:

1. Two cups of water should be brought to a boil in a medium saucepan. When the water is absorbed and the quinoa is tender, add the rinsed quinoa and a pinch of salt, lower the heat to low, cover, and simmer for 15 to 20 minutes.

2. After turning off the heat, leave the quinoa covered for five minutes. Using a fork, fluff the mixture and move it to a sizable salad dish to cool down a bit.

3. If using frozen corn, defrost the kernels by putting them in a colander and running warm water over them while the quinoa cools.

4. To the quinoa, add the chopped cilantro, diced red bell pepper, black beans, and corn.

5. To make the dressing, combine the lime juice, olive oil, ground cumin, salt, and pepper in a small bowl.

6. Drizzle the salad with the dressing and toss to thoroughly mix.

7. If needed, adjust the seasoning by tasting it.

8. Depending on personal preference, serve the salad cold or at room temperature.

73. Greek Salad with Low-Fat Feta

🕐	**Time:** 20 minutes	🍽	**Serving Size:** 4 bowls
⚖	**Prep Time:** 20 minutes	🍞	**Cook Time:** 0 minutes

Nutrition Information Per Serving (1 bowl):

Calories: 180, Carbohydrates: 10g, Saturated Fat: 3g, Protein: 7g, Fat: 12g, Sodium: 320mg, Potassium: 210mg, Fiber: 2g, Sugar: 6g, Vitamin C: 20mg, Calcium: 150mg, Iron: 1.2mg

Ingredients:

- 4 cups of romaine lettuce, chopped
- 1 medium cucumber, peeled and diced
- 2 medium tomatoes, chopped
- 1/2 red onion, thinly sliced
- 1/2 cup Kalamata olives, pitted and halved
- 1/2 cup low-fat feta cheese, crumbled
- 1/4 cup extra-virgin olive oil
- 2 tablespoons red wine vinegar
- 1 teaspoon dried oregano
- Salt and pepper to taste

Directions:

1. In a large salad bowl, combine the romaine lettuce, cucumber, tomatoes, and red onion.

2. Add the Kalamata olives and crumbled low-fat feta cheese to the bowl.

3. In a small mixing bowl, whisk together the extra-virgin olive oil, red wine vinegar, dried oregano, salt, and pepper to create the dressing.

4. Pour the dressing over the salad ingredients and toss gently to mix well and ensure all the ingredients are evenly coated.

5. Serve the salad immediately, or cover and refrigerate to chill slightly before serving.

74. Cucumber Salad with Dill and Yogurt

🕐 **Time:** 15 minutes	🍽 **Serving Size:** 4 bowls
⚖ **Prep Time:** 10 minutes	👨‍🍳 **Cook Time:** 0 minutes

Nutrition Information Per Serving (1 bowl):

Calories: 120, Carbohydrates: 10g, Saturated Fat: 0.5g, Protein: 6g, Fat: 7g, Sodium: 45mg, Potassium: 250mg, Fiber: 1g, Sugar: 5g, Vitamin C: 6mg, Calcium: 80mg, Iron: 0.7mg

Ingredients:

- 2 large cucumbers, thinly sliced
- 1 cup fat-free Greek yogurt
- 2 tablespoons fresh dill, chopped
- 1 tablespoon lemon juice
- 1 garlic clove, minced
- 1/4 teaspoon salt
- 1/4 teaspoon black pepper
- 1 tablespoon olive oil (optional for garnish)

Directions:

1. In a large mixing bowl, combine the thinly sliced cucumbers, fat-free Greek yogurt, and fresh dill.

2. Add the lemon juice and minced garlic to the mixture.

3. Season with salt and black pepper, and stir the ingredients together until the cucumbers are well coated with the yogurt and herbs.

4. If desired, drizzle with a tablespoon of olive oil for added flavor before serving.

5. Chill in the refrigerator for about 5 minutes to allow the flavors to meld together.

6. Serve the cucumber salad cold as a refreshing side dish.

75. Roasted Carrots with Honey and Thyme

🕐 **Time:** 35 minutes	🍽 **Serving Size:** 4
⚖ **Prep Time:** 5 minutes	👨‍🍳 **Cook Time:** 30 minutes

Nutrition Information Per Serving (1 serving unit):

Calories: 90, Carbohydrates: 12g, Saturated Fat: 0.5g, Protein: 1g, Fat: 4.5g, Sodium: 85mg, Potassium: 230mg, Fiber: 3g, Sugar: 7g, Vitamin C: 5mg, Calcium: 30mg, Iron: 0.5mg

Ingredients:

- 1 pound of carrots, peeled and sliced into 1/4 inch thick pieces
- 1 tablespoon of honey
- 1 tablespoon of olive oil
- 1 teaspoon of fresh thyme leaves
- Salt and pepper to taste

Directions:

1. Preheat your oven to 400°F.

2. In a large bowl, toss the carrots with the honey, olive oil, thyme leaves, salt, and pepper until they are well coated.

3. Spread the carrots out in a single layer on a baking sheet.

4. Roast in the preheated oven for about 30 minutes or until the carrots are tender and lightly caramelized, stirring halfway through the cooking time.

5. Remove from the oven and serve warm as a nutritious and delicious side dish.

76. Cauliflower Rice Pilaf

Time: 25 minutes	Serving Size: 4 bowls
Prep Time: 10 minutes	Cook Time: 15 minutes

Nutrition Information Per Serving (1 bowl):

Calories: 120, Carbohydrates: 14g, Saturated Fat: 0.5g, Protein: 4g, Fat: 6g, Sodium: 150mg, Potassium: 430mg, Fiber: 3g, Sugar: 5g, Vitamin C: 75mg, Calcium: 30mg, Iron: 1mg

Ingredients:

- 1 medium head of cauliflower
- 1 tablespoon of olive oil
- 1 small onion, finely chopped
- 2 cloves of garlic, minced
- 1/4 cup of chopped parsley
- 1/4 teaspoon of salt
- 1/4 teaspoon of black pepper
- 1/2 cup of low-sodium vegetable broth
- 1 tablespoon of lemon juice
- 1/4 cup of sliced almonds, toasted

Directions:

1. After washing, pat dry the head of cauliflower. In a food processor, pulse until it resembles rice grains after cutting into florets.

2. In a big skillet over medium heat, warm up the olive oil. Add the chopped onion and minced garlic, and cook for about 3 minutes, or until the onion becomes transparent.

3. Add the cauliflower rice and simmer, stirring often, for an additional five minutes.

4. Stir in the black pepper, salt, and chopped parsley.

5. After adding the lemon juice and low-sodium vegetable broth, cover the skillet. Simmer the cauliflower for 5 to 7 minutes, or until it is soft and the liquid has been absorbed.

6. Take off the heat and carefully mix in the almond slices that have been roasted.

7. Serve warm as a tasty and nutritious side dish to go with a range of main dishes.

77. Broccoli Salad with Almonds and Cranberries

Time: 20 minutes	Serving Size: 4 bowls
Prep Time: 15 minutes	Cook Time: 0 minutes

Nutrition Information Per Serving (1 bowl):

Calories: 110, Carbohydrates: 15g, Saturated Fat 1g, Protein: 4g, Fat: 5g, Sodium: 65mg, Potassium: 350mg, Fiber: 3g, Sugar: 7g, Vitamin C: 101mg, Calcium: 55mg, Iron: 1mg

Ingredients:

- 4 cups of fresh broccoli florets
- 1/4 cup of sliced almonds, toasted
- 1/4 cup of dried cranberries
- 1 tablespoon of apple cider vinegar
- 1 tablespoon of honey
- Salt and pepper to taste
- 1/4 cup of fat-free mayonnaise

Directions:

1. Begin by washing the fresh broccoli florets and cutting them into bite-sized pieces if necessary

2. In a large salad bowl, combine the broccoli, toasted sliced almonds, and dried cranberries.

3. In a small bowl, whisk together the fat-free mayonnaise, apple cider vinegar, and honey until smooth.

4. Pour the dressing over the broccoli mixture and toss to coat evenly.

5. Season the salad with salt and pepper to your liking.

6. Let the salad sit in the refrigerator for about 5 minutes to allow the flavors to combine.

7. Serve the broccoli salad chilled as a nutritious and flavorful side dish.

78. Green Bean Almondine

⏰ Time: 25 minutes	🍽 Serving Size: 4
⚖ Prep Time: 10 minutes	👨‍🍳 Cook Time: 15 minutes

Nutrition Information Per Serving (1 serving unit):

Calories: 90, Carbohydrates: 10g, Saturated Fat: 0.1g, Protein: 3g, Fat: 5g, Sodium: 30mg, Potassium: 240mg, Fiber: 3g, Sugar: 4g, Vitamin C: 12mg, Calcium: 55mg, Iron: 1.2mg

Ingredients:

- 1 pound fresh green beans, trimmed
- 1 tablespoon slivered almonds
- 1 teaspoon extra virgin olive oil
- 1 tablespoon lemon juice
- Salt and pepper to taste
- 1 clove garlic, minced

Directions:

1. In a steamer basket set over boiling water, steam the green beans for approximately five minutes, or until they are crisp but still soft.

2. In a dry skillet over medium heat, toast the slivered almonds until fragrant and golden brown, turning often to avoid burning, while the green beans are steaming. This ought to take three minutes or so. Take off the heat and place aside.

3. Heat the olive oil in a big skillet over medium heat. Add the minced garlic and cook until aromatic, about 30 seconds.

4. Toss to coat the steaming green beans after adding them to the skillet with the garlic. Simmer for two more minutes.

5. After taking off the heat, pour the lemon juice over the green beans. Add salt and pepper to taste and toss the green beans with the roasted almonds.

6. Warm up and enjoy as a light and nutritious side dish.

79. Sweet Corn and Tomato Salad

⏰ Time: 20 minutes	🍽 Serving Size: 4 bowls
⚖ Prep Time: 10 minutes	👨‍🍳 Cook Time: 10 minutes

Nutrition Information Per Serving (1 bowl):

Calories: 125, Carbohydrates: 27g, Saturated Fat: 0.5g, Protein: 4g, Fat: 1.5g, Sodium: 15mg, Potassium: 394mg, Fiber: 3g, Sugar: 9g, Vitamin C: 12mg, Calcium: 14mg, Iron: 0.7mg

Ingredients:

- 4 ears of fresh sweet corn, husks and silks removed
- 1 cup cherry tomatoes, halved
- 1/4 cup red onion, finely chopped
- 1/4 cup fresh basil leaves, thinly sliced
- 2 tablespoons white wine vinegar
- 1 tablespoon extra-virgin olive oil
- 1/4 teaspoon salt
- 1/8 teaspoon freshly ground black pepper

Directions:

1. Pour water into a big saucepan and heat it until it boils. When the water reaches a rolling boil, carefully add the corn ears and cook until the kernels are soft, about 10 minutes.

2. When the corn is cool enough to handle, remove it from the pot. After slicing the kernels from the cobs, transfer them to a big salad bowl.

3. Add the thinly sliced basil leaves, finely chopped red onion, and split cherry tomatoes to the bowl.

4. To make the dressing, combine the extra-virgin olive oil, white wine vinegar, salt, and freshly ground black pepper in a small bowl.

5. Pour the dressing over the corn and tomato mixture, then toss lightly to incorporate everything together.

6. To help the flavors combine, place the salad in the refrigerator for a minimum of 10 minutes.

7. As a light and pleasant side dish, serve the salad cold.

80. Mediterranean Chickpea Salad

	Time: 15 minutes		Serving Size: 4 bowls
	Prep Time: 15 minutes		Cook Time: 0 minutes

Nutrition Information Per Serving (1 bowl):

Calories: 180, Carbohydrates: 30g, Saturated Fat: 0.5g, Protein: 7g, Fat: 4g, Sodium: 300mg, Potassium: 360mg, Fiber: 8g, Sugar: 5g, Vitamin C: 8mg, Calcium: 80mg, Iron: 2.5mg

Ingredients:

- 2 cups canned chickpeas, drained and rinsed
- 1 cup cherry tomatoes, halved
- 1 cup cucumber, diced
- 1/2 cup red onion, finely chopped
- 1/4 cup fresh parsley, chopped
- 1/4 cup fresh mint, chopped
- Juice of 1 lemon
- 1 tablespoon extra-virgin olive oil
- 1 teaspoon dried oregano
- Salt and pepper to taste

Directions:

1. Drained and rinsed chickpeas, diced cucumber, finely chopped red onion, chopped fresh parsley, and chopped fresh mint should all be combined in a big mixing basin.

2. To make a simple dressing, combine the extra virgin olive oil, dried oregano, and lemon juice in a small bowl.

3. Drizzle the chickpea mixture with the dressing, then toss gently to coat all the ingredients.

4. To taste, add more salt and pepper to the salad. As needed, adjust the seasoning.

5. Before serving, let the salad sit for five to ten minutes so the flavors can mingle.

6. The Mediterranean Chickpea Salad is a tasty and nourishing side dish that may be served cold or room temperature.

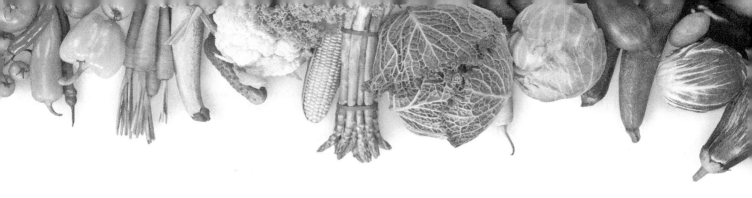

CHAPTER 10: DESSERTS

81. Baked Apples with Cinnamon and Nutmeg

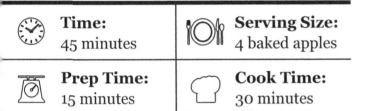

	Time: 45 minutes		Serving Size: 4 baked apples
	Prep Time: 15 minutes		Cook Time: 30 minutes

Nutrition Information Per Serving (1 baked apple):

Calories: 190, Carbohydrates: 51g, Saturated Fat: 0.2g, Protein: 0.5g, Fat: 0.4g, Sodium: 2mg, Potassium: 194mg, Fiber: 5g, Sugar: 43g, Vitamin C: 8.4mg, Calcium: 20mg, Iron: 0.3mg

Ingredients:

- 4 large apples, such as Fuji or Gala
- 1/4 cup brown sugar
- 1/2 teaspoon ground cinnamon
- 1/4 teaspoon ground nutmeg
- 1/2 cup apple juice or water
- 1/4 teaspoon vanilla extract

Directions:

1. Preheat your oven to 350°F.

2. Core the apples and place them in a baking dish that comfortably fits all four.

3. In a small bowl, mix together the brown sugar, ground cinnamon, and ground nutmeg.

4. Fill each apple's hollowed core with the sugar and spice mixture.

5. In a separate bowl, combine the apple juice (or water) with the vanilla extract, then pour this liquid into the bottom of the baking dish around the apples.

6. Bake in the preheated oven for 30 minutes, or until the apples are tender when pierced with a fork.

7. Carefully remove the apples from the oven and allow them to cool slightly before serving.

82. Avocado Chocolate Mousse

	Time: 10 minutes		Serving Size: 2 glass
	Prep Time: 10 minutes		Cook Time: 0 minutes

Nutrition Information Per Serving (1 glass):

Calories: 300, Carbohydrates: 35g, Saturated Fat: 3g, Protein: 4g, Fat: 19g, Sodium: 35mg, Potassium: 487mg, Fiber: 8g, Sugar: 20g, Vitamin C: 10mg, Calcium: 20mg, Iron: 1.2mg

Ingredients:

- 2 ripe avocados, peeled and pitted
- 1/4 cup unsweetened cocoa powder
- 1/4 cup honey or maple syrup (for a low-fat option, use a suitable sweetener)
- 1/2 teaspoon pure vanilla extract
- A pinch of salt
- Fresh berries for garnish (optional)

Directions:

1. Place the peeled and pitted avocados in a food processor or blender.
2. Add the unsweetened cocoa powder, honey or maple syrup, pure vanilla extract, and a pinch of salt to the avocados.
3. Blend the mixture until smooth and creamy, scraping down the sides as needed to ensure all ingredients are well incorporated.
4. Taste the mousse and adjust the sweetness if necessary.
5. Divide the mousse into serving dishes and refrigerate for at least 30 minutes to chill and set.
6. Before serving, garnish with fresh berries if desired for added flavor and a pop of color.
7. Enjoy this rich and creamy Avocado Chocolate Mousse as a delightful, pancreatitis-friendly dessert.

83. Pineapple Sorbet

⏰ **Time:** 2 hours 10 min	🍽 **Serving Size:** 4 cups
⚖ **Prep Time:** 10 minutes	👨‍🍳 **Cook Time:** 2 hours

Nutrition Information Per Serving (1 cup):

Calories: 75, Carbohydrates: 19g, Saturated Fat: 0g, Protein: 0g, Fat: 0g, Sodium: 1mg, Potassium: 120mg, Fiber: 1g, Sugar: 14g, Vitamin C: 40mg, Calcium: 15mg, Iron: 0.2mg

Ingredients:

- Juice of 1 lime
- 1 tablespoon honey (optional, for added sweetness)
- 1 large pineapple
- Fresh mint leaves for garnish (optional)

Directions:

1. Peel the pineapple and chop it into chunks, removing the core.
2. Place the pineapple chunks into a blender or food processor.
3. Add the juice of 1 lime to the blender, along with the honey if desired for extra sweetness.
4. Blend the mixture until smooth.
5. Pour the blended pineapple into an airtight container and freeze for about 2 hours, or until it starts to solidify around the edges.
6. Remove the container from the freezer and stir the sorbet vigorously with a fork, breaking up any frozen sections.
7. Return the sorbet to the freezer and repeat the stirring process every 30 minutes for about 2 hours, or until the sorbet is fully frozen and has a smooth consistency.
8. Serve the pineapple sorbet in bowls, garnished with fresh mint leaves if desired.

84. Almond and Date Truffles

⏱ **Time:** 15 minutes	🍴 **Serving Size:** 10 truffles
⚖ **Prep Time:** 15 minutes	👨‍🍳 **Cook Time:** 0 minutes

Nutrition Information Per Serving (1 truffle):

Calories: 95, Carbohydrates: 18g, Saturated Fat: 0.1g, Protein: 2g, Fat: 2.5g, Sodium: 1mg, Potassium: 210mg, Fiber: 3g, Sugar: 14g, Vitamin C: 0.1mg, Calcium: 20mg, Iron: 0.5mg

Ingredients:

- 1 cup pitted dates
- 1/2 cup raw almonds
- 1/4 teaspoon ground cinnamon
- 1/8 teaspoon salt
- 1 teaspoon almond extract
- 2 tablespoons unsweetened shredded coconut for coating

Directions:

1. Place the pitted dates and raw almonds into a food processor.
2. Add the ground cinnamon, salt, and almond extract to the mixture.
3. Process until the mixture sticks together and forms a dough-like consistency.
4. Take a tablespoon of the mixture and roll it into a ball between your palms.
5. Roll the truffle balls in unsweetened shredded coconut to coat them evenly.
6. Place the truffles on a plate and chill in the refrigerator for at least an hour to firm up.
7. Serve the Almond and Date Truffles chilled as a sweet, yet healthy dessert option for those managing pancreatitis.

85. Peach and Raspberry Crisp

⏱ **Time:** 45 minutes	🍴 **Serving Size:** 6
⚖ **Prep Time:** 15 minutes	👨‍🍳 **Cook Time:** 30 minutes

Nutrition Information Per Serving (1 serving unit):

Calories: 150, Carbohydrates: 31g, Saturated Fat: 0.5g, Protein: 2g, Fat: 2g, Sodium: 10mg, Potassium: 200mg, Fiber: 4g, Sugar: 22g, Vitamin C: 12mg, Calcium: 20mg, Iron: 0.7mg

Ingredients:

- 4 medium peaches, pitted and sliced
- 1 cup fresh raspberries
- 2 tablespoons granulated sugar or a suitable sugar substitute
- 1/4 teaspoon ground cinnamon
- 1/4 teaspoon ground nutmeg
- 1/2 cup rolled oats
- 1/4 cup almond flour
- 2 tablespoons cold water
- Cooking spray (for the baking dish)

Directions:

1. Preheat your oven to 350°F (175°C).
2. In a large bowl, mix the sliced peaches, raspberries, sugar, cinnamon, and nutmeg until the fruit is evenly coated.
3. Spray a baking dish with cooking spray and transfer the fruit mixture into the dish.
4. In a separate bowl, combine the rolled oats and almond flour.
5. Sprinkle the oat and almond flour mixture over the fruit.
6. Drizzle the cold water evenly over the top of the oat mixture.

7. Place the baking dish in the oven and bake for 30 minutes, or until the topping is golden brown and the fruit is bubbly.

8. Remove from the oven and let it cool slightly before serving.

86. Coconut Rice Pudding

⏰ **Time:** 40 minutes	🍽 **Serving Size:** 6 cups
⚖ **Prep Time:** 10 minutes	👨‍🍳 **Cook Time:** 30 minutes

Nutrition Information Per Serving (1 cup):

Calories: 215, Carbohydrates: 38g, Saturated Fat: 5g, Protein: 4g, Fat: 5g, Sodium: 50mg, Potassium: 142mg, Fiber: 1g, Sugar: 12g, Vitamin C: 0.8mg, Calcium: 20mg, Iron: 0.4mg

Ingredients:

- 1 cup jasmine or basmati rice
- 1 can (13.5 ounces) light coconut milk
- 2 cups water
- 1/4 cup sugar
- 1/4 teaspoon salt
- 1/2 teaspoon vanilla extract
- Ground cinnamon for garnish (optional)

Directions:

1. Rinse the rice under cold water until the water runs clear.

2. In a medium-sized pot, combine the rinsed rice, light coconut milk, water, sugar, and salt.

3. Bring the mixture to a boil over medium-high heat, then reduce the heat to low.

4. Cover the pot and simmer for about 30 minutes, or until the rice is tender and the liquid has been absorbed.

5. Remove from heat and stir in the vanilla extract.

6. Allow the pudding to cool slightly before serving, or chill in the refrigerator if preferred cold.

7. Serve the coconut rice pudding in individual bowls, sprinkled with ground cinnamon as a garnish if desired.

87. Strawberry Banana Smoothie Bowl

⏰ **Time:** 10 minutes	🍽 **Serving Size:** 2 bowls
⚖ **Prep Time:** 10 minutes	👨‍🍳 **Cook Time:** 0 minutes

Nutrition Information Per Serving (1 bowl):

Calories: 185, Carbohydrates: 44g, Saturated Fat: 0.2g, Protein: 3g, Fat: 1g, Sodium: 3mg, Potassium: 633mg, Fiber: 7g, Sugar: 28g, Vitamin C: 94mg, Calcium: 20mg, Iron: 0.6mg

Ingredients:

- 1 cup strawberries, hulled and frozen
- 1/2 cup unsweetened almond milk
- 1/2 teaspoon honey (optional, depending on your dietary needs)
- 1 large banana, sliced and frozen
- Fresh strawberries, for garnish
- Banana slices, for garnish
- A sprinkle of chia seeds, for garnish

Directions:

1. Place the frozen banana slices and frozen strawberries into a blender.

2. Add the unsweetened almond milk and honey (if using) to the blender.

3. Blend on high until the mixture is smooth and creamy, stopping to scrape down the sides as necessary.

4. Pour the smoothie mixture into two bowls.

5. Garnish with fresh strawberry slices, banana slices, and a sprinkle of chia seeds.

6. Serve immediately and enjoy your refreshing Strawberry Banana Smoothie Bowl!

88. Blueberry Oatmeal Cookies

⏰ **Time:** 35 minutes	🍽️ **Serving Size:** 12 cookies
⚖️ **Prep Time:** 15 minutes	👨‍🍳 **Cook Time:** 20 minutes

Nutrition Information Per Serving (1 cookie):

Calories: 110, Carbohydrates: 18g, Saturated Fat: 0.5g, Protein: 3g, Fat: 3g, Sodium: 70mg, Potassium: 85mg, Fiber: 2g, Sugar: 9g, Vitamin C: 1mg, Calcium: 16mg, Iron: 0.7mg

Ingredients:

- 1 cup rolled oats
- 3/4 cup whole wheat flour
- 1/2 teaspoon baking soda
- 1/4 teaspoon salt
- 1/4 cup unsweetened applesauce
- 1/4 cup honey or maple syrup
- 1 large egg
- 1 teaspoon vanilla extract
- 1/2 cup fresh blueberries

Directions:

1. Preheat your oven to 350°F (175°C).

2. In a large bowl, whisk together the rolled oats, whole wheat flour, baking soda, and salt.

3. In a separate bowl, mix the unsweetened applesauce, honey or maple syrup, egg, and

vanilla extract until well combined.

4. Gradually add the wet ingredients to the dry ingredients, stirring until just combined.

5. Gently fold in the fresh blueberries.

6. Drop tablespoonfuls of the dough onto a baking sheet lined with parchment paper, spacing them about 2 inches apart.

7. Bake for 18-20 minutes, or until the edges are golden brown.

8. Allow the cookies to cool on the baking sheet for 5 minutes before transferring them to a wire rack to cool completely.

9. Serve and enjoy your Blueberry Oatmeal Cookies!

89. Mango and Sticky Rice

⏰ **Time:** 45 minutes	🍽️ **Serving Size:** 4
⚖️ **Prep Time:** 15 minutes	👨‍🍳 **Cook Time:** 30 minutes

Nutrition Information Per Serving (1 serving unit):

Calories: 270, Carbohydrates: 60g, Saturated Fat: 1g, Protein: 4g, Fat: 1g, Sodium: 15mg, Potassium: 170mg, Fiber: 2g, Sugar: 15g, Vitamin C: 20mg, Calcium: 10mg, Iron: 0.5mg

Ingredients:

- 1 cup Thai sticky rice (also known as glutinous rice)
- 1 ripe mango, peeled and sliced
- 1 cup canned light coconut milk
- 1/4 cup granulated sugar
- 1/4 teaspoon salt
- 1/2 teaspoon cornstarch
- 1 tablespoon water
- Toasted sesame seeds, for garnish (optional)

Directions:

1. Rinse the sticky rice in cold water until the water runs clear. Soak the rice in water for at least an hour or overnight.

2. Drain the rice and steam in a bamboo steamer or a pot with a tight-fitting lid for about 20-30 minutes, or until tender.

3. While the rice is cooking, combine the coconut milk, sugar, and salt in a saucepan. Heat over medium heat until the sugar dissolves. Do not boil.

4. In a small bowl, dissolve the cornstarch in the tablespoon of water and add to the coconut milk mixture, stirring well to thicken slightly.

5. Once the rice is cooked, transfer it to a bowl and pour 3/4 of the coconut milk mixture over the rice. Stir well and let it sit for a few minutes to allow the flavors to meld.

6. Serve the sticky rice with sliced mango on top. Drizzle the remaining coconut milk mixture over the rice and mango.

7. Garnish with toasted sesame seeds if desired.

8. Enjoy your Mango and Sticky Rice, a classic dessert with a pancreatitis-friendly twist!

90. Chocolate-Dipped Strawberries

	Time: 30 minutes		**Serving Size:** 4 strawberries
	Prep Time: 10 minutes		**Cook Time:** 20 minutes

Nutrition Information Per Serving (1 strawberry):

Calories: 150, Carbohydrates: 20g, Saturated Fat: 2g, Protein: 1g, Fat: 8g, Sodium: 20mg, Potassium: 160mg, Fiber: 3g, Sugar: 15g, Vitamin C: 50mg, Calcium: 15mg, Iron: 0.5mg

Ingredients:

- 100g dark chocolate (at least 70% cocoa), broken into pieces
- 1 tsp coconut oil
- 16 large fresh strawberries, leaves intact
- Optional: a pinch of sea salt

Directions:

1. Line a baking sheet with parchment paper.

2. Rinse the strawberries and pat them dry with paper towels, ensuring they are completely dry.

3. In a microwave-safe bowl, combine the dark chocolate pieces and coconut oil.

4. Microwave in 30-second intervals, stirring between each, until the chocolate is fully melted and smooth.

5. Holding a strawberry by the leaves, dip it into the melted chocolate, letting the excess drip back into the bowl.

6. Place the chocolate-dipped strawberry onto the lined baking sheet. Repeat with the remaining strawberries.

7. If desired, sprinkle a tiny pinch of sea salt on each strawberry before the chocolate sets.

8. Place the baking sheet in the refrigerator for about 20 minutes, or until the chocolate is firm.

9. Serve the chocolate-dipped strawberries immediately, or store them in an airtight container in the refrigerator for up to 24 hours

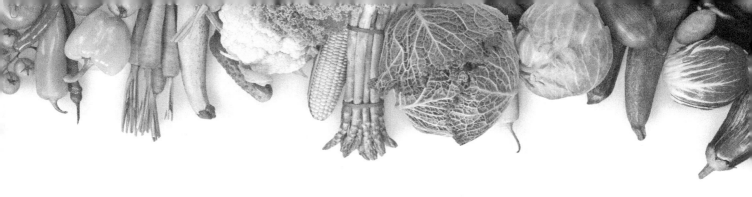

CHAPTER 11: BEVERAGES

91. Beetroot and Carrot Juice

 Time: 15 minutes	 Serving Size: 2 glasses
Prep Time: 5 minutes	Cook Time: 10 minutes

Nutrition Information Per Serving (1 glass):

Calories: 95, Carbohydrates: 22g, Saturated Fat: 0g, Protein: 2g, Fat: 0.3g, Sodium: 77mg, Potassium: 687mg, Fiber: 5.6g, Sugar: 9g, Vitamin C: 10mg, Calcium: 39mg, Iron: 1.1mg

Ingredients:

- 1 medium beetroot, peeled and chopped
- 2 medium carrots, peeled and chopped
- 1 apple, cored and sliced
- 1-inch piece of fresh ginger, peeled
- 1 cup water or coconut water
- Ice cubes (optional)

Directions:

1. Prepare the beetroot and carrots by thoroughly washing, peeling, and chopping them into small pieces that can fit into your juicer.
2. Core the apple and cut it into slices. Peel the ginger.
3. Combine the beetroot, carrots, apple, and ginger in the juicer.
4. Add water or coconut water to the juicer to help extract the juice, if needed.
5. Turn on the juicer and push the ingredients through, collecting the juice in a glass or jug.
6. If desired, add ice cubes to the juice for a chilled beverage.
7. Stir the juice well before serving to ensure all flavors are well combined.
8. Pour the juice into glasses and enjoy immediately for the best taste and nutrient content.

92. Cucumber Mint Water

 Time: 5 minutes	 Serving Size: 4 glasses
Prep Time: 5 minutes	Cook Time: 0 minutes

Nutrition Information Per Serving (1 glass):

Calories: 5, Carbohydrates: 1g, Saturated Fat: 0g, Protein: 0g, Fat: 0g, Sodium: 6mg, Potassium: 76mg, Fiber: 0.5g, Sugar: 0.4g, Vitamin C: 2.4mg, Calcium: 14mg, Iron: 0.2mg

Ingredients:

- 1 medium cucumber, thinly sliced
- 8 cups of cold water
- 1/4 cup fresh mint leaves
- Ice cubes (optional)

Directions:

1. Rinse the cucumber and mint leaves thoroughly under cold water.

2. In a large pitcher, combine the sliced cucumber and fresh mint leaves.

3. Fill the pitcher with 8 cups of cold water, stirring gently to distribute the flavors.

4. Refrigerate the mixture for at least 1 hour to allow the flavors to infuse. You can let it sit for up to 4 hours for a stronger flavor.

5. Before serving, stir the water again and add ice cubes if desired for a chilled, refreshing beverage.

6. Pour the cucumber mint water into glasses, being sure to include a few cucumber slices and mint leaves in each glass for garnish.

93. Lemon and Ginger Infusion

⏱ Time: 10 minutes	🍽 Serving Size: 1 cup
⏲ Prep Time: 5 minutes	👨‍🍳 Cook Time: 5 minutes

Nutrition Information Per Serving (1 cup):

Calories: 12, Carbohydrates: 3g, Saturated Fat: 0g, Protein: 0g, Fat: 0g, Sodium: 1mg, Potassium: 49mg, Fiber: 0.6g, Sugar: 0.6g, Vitamin C: 10mg, Calcium: 11mg, Iron: 0.1mg

Ingredients:

- 1 cup water
- 1 inch fresh ginger root, peeled and thinly sliced
- 1/2 lemon, juiced
- 1 teaspoon honey (optional)

Directions:

1. Bring 1 cup of water to a boil in a small pot or saucepan.

2. Once the water is boiling, add the sliced ginger root to the pot and reduce the heat to a low simmer.

3. Allow the ginger to steep in the simmering water for about 5 minutes.

4. Remove the pot from the heat and strain the ginger pieces from the water, pouring the infused water into a mug.

5. Squeeze the juice of half a lemon into the ginger-infused water, stirring to combine.

6. If a touch of sweetness is desired, stir in 1 teaspoon of honey until it is fully dissolved.

7. Enjoy the Lemon and Ginger Infusion warm, ideally sipping slowly to savor the flavors and aid digestion.

94. Berry and Spinach Smoothie

⏱ Time: 10 minutes	🍽 Serving Size: 1 glass
⏲ Prep Time: 5 minutes	👨‍🍳 Cook Time: 5 minutes

Nutrition Information Per Serving (1 glass):

Calories: 120, Carbohydrates: 25g, Saturated Fat: 0.1g, Protein: 3g, Fat: 1g, Sodium: 50mg, Potassium: 400mg, Fiber: 4g, Sugar: 15g, Vitamin C: 24mg, Calcium: 30mg, Iron: 0.7mg

Ingredients:

- 1/2 cup mixed berries (strawberries, blueberries, raspberries), fresh or frozen
- 1 cup baby spinach leaves, washed
- 1/2 banana, sliced
- 1 cup unsweetened almond milk
- 1 tablespoon honey (optional, depending on your diet plan and doctor's advice)
- 1/2 cup ice cubes (optional)

Directions:

1. In a blender, combine the mixed berries, banana, and baby spinach leaves.

2. Add the unsweetened almond milk to the blender. If you're including honey for sweetness, add it now.

3. Blend on high speed until the mixture is smooth and creamy. If the smoothie is too thick, you can add a little more almond milk to reach your desired consistency.

4. If you prefer a colder smoothie, add ice cubes to the blender and blend again until the ice is fully incorporated.

5. Pour the smoothie into a glass and serve immediately for the freshest taste and most nutrients.

95. Almond Milk Latte

⏰ **Time:** 10 minutes	🍽 **Serving Size:** 1 cup
⚖ **Prep Time:** 5 minutes	👨‍🍳 **Cook Time:** 5 minutes

Nutrition Information Per Serving (1 cup):

Calories: 50, Carbohydrates: 2g, Saturated Fat: 0g, Protein: 1g, Fat: 4g, Sodium: 150mg, Potassium: 50mg, Fiber: 1g, Sugar: 0g, Vitamin C: 0mg, Calcium: 450mg, Iron: 0.5mg

Ingredients:

- 1 cup unsweetened almond milk
- 1 shot of espresso or 1/4 cup strong brewed coffee
- Optional: a dash of cinnamon or nutmeg
- Optional: sweetener of choice (e.g., stevia, monk fruit sweetener)

Directions:

1. Begin by heating the almond milk in a small saucepan over medium heat. Heat until the milk is hot but not boiling, stirring occasionally to prevent a skin from forming on the surface.

2. While the almond milk is heating, prepare your espresso or strong brewed coffee. If you're using a coffee maker, ensure it's set to brew a concentrated cup.

3. Once the almond milk is hot, froth it using a milk frother or by whisking vigorously to create a light foam.

4. Pour the espresso or coffee into a large mug, and then gently add the frothed almond milk.

5. If desired, sprinkle a dash of cinnamon or nutmeg on top for added flavor, and sweeten to taste with your preferred sweetener.

6. Serve the almond milk latte immediately, stirring gently to combine the flavors if you've added spices or sweetener.

96. Watermelon and Lime Cooler

⏰ **Time:** 15 minutes	🍽 **Serving Size:** 1 glass
⚖ **Prep Time:** 10 minutes	👨‍🍳 **Cook Time:** 5 minutes

Nutrition Information Per Serving (1 glass):

Calories: 100, Carbohydrates: 25g, Saturated Fat: 0g, Protein: 2g, Fat: 0.5g, Sodium: 5mg, Potassium: 300mg, Fiber: 1g, Sugar: 20g, Vitamin C: 25mg, Calcium: 20mg, Iron: 0.4mg

Ingredients:

- 2 cups seedless watermelon, cubed
- Juice of 1 lime
- 1 cup ice cubes
- Optional: mint leaves for garnish
- Optional: 1 teaspoon honey or sweetener of choice

Directions:

1. Place the watermelon cubes into a blender and blend until smooth.
2. Strain the watermelon through a fine mesh sieve into a large bowl, discarding the solid bits to ensure a smooth drink.
3. Pour the strained watermelon juice back into the blender. Add the freshly squeezed lime juice and ice cubes.
4. If you prefer a sweeter taste, add honey or your choice of sweetener. Blend until the mixture is slushy.
5. Pour the cooler into a glass and garnish with mint leaves if desired.
6. Serve immediately for a refreshing and hydrating beverage that's gentle on the pancreas.

Ingredients:

- 1 peach, pitted and sliced
- 1 bag of herbal tea (caffeine-free)
- 1 cup of boiling water
- Ice cubes
- Fresh mint leaves for garnish (optional)
- Honey or sweetener of choice (optional)

Directions:

1. Place the peach slices in a heatproof pitcher or bowl.
2. Steep the herbal tea bag in 1 cup of boiling water for about 5 minutes.
3. Remove the tea bag and pour the hot tea over the peach slices. Let it infuse for about 10 minutes.
4. Strain the tea to remove the peach slices and any loose tea leaves. If you prefer a sweeter drink, stir in honey or your chosen sweetener while the tea is still warm.
5. Fill a tall glass with ice cubes and pour the peach-infused tea over the ice.
6. Garnish with fresh mint leaves if desired.
7. Enjoy your refreshing Peach Iced Tea, perfect for a warm day or a soothing evening drink.

97. Peach Iced Tea

⏰ **Time:** 20 minutes	🍽 **Serving Size:** 1 glass
⚖ **Prep Time:** 5 minutes	👨‍🍳 **Cook Time:** 15 minutes

Nutrition Information Per Serving (1 glass):

Calories: 60, Carbohydrates: 15g, Saturated Fat: 0g, Protein: 1g, Fat: 0g, Sodium: 10mg, Potassium: 75mg, Fiber: 1g, Sugar: 14g, Vitamin C: 5mg, Calcium: 10mg, Iron: 0.2mg

98. Coconut Water Smoothie

⏰ **Time:** 10 minutes	🍽 **Serving Size:** 1 glass
⚖ **Prep Time:** 5 minutes	👨‍🍳 **Cook Time:** 0 minutes

Nutrition Information Per Serving (1 glass):

Calories: 150, Carbohydrates: 19g, Saturated Fat: 0g, Protein: 2g, Fat: 0.5g, Sodium: 25mg, Potassium: 600mg, Fiber: 3g, Sugar: 12g, Vitamin C: 10mg, Calcium: 60mg, Iron: 0.3mg

Ingredients:

- 1 cup coconut water
- 1/2 banana
- 1/2 cup frozen pineapple chunks
- 1/2 cup frozen mango chunks
- Optional: A handful of spinach leaves for added nutrients

Directions:

1. Pour 1 cup of coconut water into a blender.
2. Add the 1/2 banana, 1/2 cup of frozen pineapple chunks, and 1/2 cup of frozen mango chunks to the blender.
3. If you choose, add a handful of fresh spinach leaves for an extra nutritional boost.
4. Blend on high speed until all the ingredients are well combined and the smoothie has a creamy consistency.
5. Pour the smoothie into a glass and serve immediately for a refreshing, tropical beverage that's suitable for a pancreatitis-friendly diet.

Directions:

1. Heat the water in a small saucepan over medium heat until it begins to simmer. Do not let it come to a boil to preserve the delicate flavors and nutrients of the honey and lemon.
2. While the water is heating, squeeze the juice of half a lemon into a cup.
3. Add the honey to the cup, adjusting the amount to taste if necessary.
4. Once the water has reached a simmer, pour it over the lemon and honey in the cup.
5. Stir the mixture until the honey has fully dissolved into the water.
6. Garnish with a slice of lemon on the rim of the cup if desired.
7. Enjoy the hot lemon and honey beverage while warm for a soothing and comforting drink that's suitable for a pancreatitis-friendly diet.

99. Hot Lemon and Honey

⏰ Time: 10 minutes	🍽 Serving Size: 1 cup
⚖ Prep Time: 5 minutes	👨‍🍳 Cook Time: 5 minutes

Nutrition Information Per Serving (1 cup):

Calories: 60, Carbohydrates: 17g, Saturated Fat: 0g, Protein: 0.3g, Fat: 0g, Sodium: 5mg, Potassium: 31mg, Fiber: 0.2g, Sugar: 16g, Vitamin C: 11mg, Calcium: 6mg, Iron: 0.1mg

Ingredients:

- 1 cup of water
- Juice of 1/2 a lemon
- 1 tablespoon of honey
- A slice of lemon for garnish (optional)

100. Pomegranate Spritzer

⏰ Time: 5 minutes	🍽 Serving Size: 1 glass
⚖ Prep Time: 3 minutes	👨‍🍳 Cook Time: 2 minutes

Nutrition Information Per Serving (1 glass):

Calories: 90, Carbohydrates: 22g, Saturated Fat: 0g, Protein: 0g, Fat: 0g, Sodium: 13mg, Potassium: 240mg, Fiber: 0.2g, Sugar: 21g, Vitamin C: 0.1mg, Calcium: 16mg, Iron: 0.1mg

Ingredients:

- 1/2 cup pomegranate juice, no sugar added
- 1/2 cup sparkling water
- Ice cubes
- Lemon wedge for garnish
- Fresh mint leaves for garnish (optional)

Directions:

1. Fill a glass halfway with ice cubes.

2. Pour 1/2 cup of pomegranate juice over the ice.

3. Top the pomegranate juice with 1/2 cup of sparkling water, creating a fizzy effect.

4. Gently stir the mixture with a spoon to combine the juice and sparkling water.

5. Garnish with a lemon wedge and, if desired, a few fresh mint leaves for a refreshing aroma and taste.

6. Serve the pomegranate spritzer immediately for a light and rejuvenating beverage suitable for those managing pancreatitis.

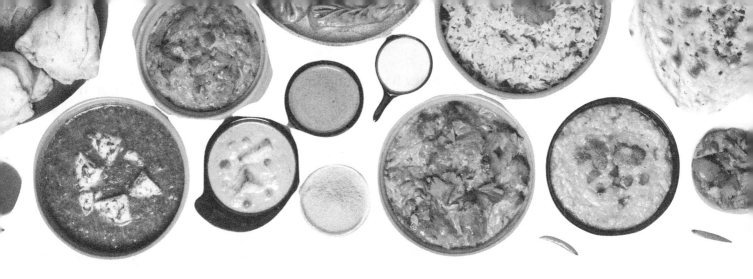

CHAPTER 12: 28-DAY MEAL PREP PLAN

DAY	BREAKFAST	LUNCH	SNACK OR APPETIZER	DINNER
1	Apple-Cinnamon Oat Porridge	Cauliflower Steak with Herb Sauce	Carrot and Zucchini Sticks with Baba Ganoush	Roast Beef with Root Vegetables
2	Quinoa Breakfast Bowl with Berries	Turkey Meatballs in Tomato Sauce	Baked Sweet Potato Fries	Baked Salmon with Dill and Lemon
3	Pumpkin Spice Oatmeal	Vegetable Minestrone	Cucumber Rounds with Hummus	Beef Stir Fry with Broccoli and Bell Peppers
4	Spinach and Feta Egg Muffins	Stuffed Bell Peppers with Quinoa	Fruit Salad with Mint and Lime Dressing	Sea Bass with Mediterranean Vegetables
5	Banana and Walnut Smoothie	Chicken and Rice Soup	Baked Sweet Potato Fries	Tofu Scramble with Vegetables
6	Greek Yogurt with Honey and Almonds	Vegan Chili with Sweet Potato	Carrot and Zucchini Sticks with Baba Ganoush	Pork Chops with Peach Salsa

7	Sweet Potato and Kale Hash	Tomato Basil Soup	Melon and Prosciutto Bites	Lemon Herb Roasted Chicken
8	Apple-Cinnamon Oat Porridge	Italian Sausage and Tortellini Soup	Rice Paper Rolls with Avocado and Mango	Turkey Burger with Avocado
9	Sweet Potato and Chickpea Stew	Eggplant Parmesan Casserole	Sliced Apples with Almond Butter	Shrimp and Asparagus Stir Fry
10	Cottage Cheese with Pineapple Chunks	Pea and Ham Hock Soup	Tomato Bruschetta on Whole Grain Bread	Grilled Tilapia with Mango Salsa
11	Pumpkin Spice Oatmeal	Cauliflower Steak with Herb Sauce	Veggie Nori Rolls	Meatloaf with Turkey and Quinoa
12	Scrambled Tofu with Spinach and Tomatoes	Broccoli and Potato Soup	Tomato Bruschetta on Whole Grain Bread	Slow Cooker Pulled Pork
13	Pear and Ginger Overnight Oats	Sweet Potato and Chickpea Stew	Baked Kale Chips	Chicken Fajitas with Whole Wheat Tortillas
14	Cottage Cheese with Pineapple Chunks	Spicy Black Bean Soup	Rice Paper Rolls with Avocado and Mango	Steamed Brown Rice
15	Apple-Cinnamon Oat Porridge	Vegan Shepherd's Pie	Carrot and Zucchini Sticks with Baba Ganoush	Chicken Cacciatore
16	Quinoa Breakfast Bowl with Berries	Italian Sausage and Tortellini Soup	Baked Sweet Potato Fries	Roast Beef with Root Vegetables
17	Sweet Potato and Chickpea Stew	Cauliflower Steak with Herb Sauce	Cucumber Rounds with Hummus	Beef Stir Fry with Broccoli and Bell Peppers

18	Spinach and Feta Egg Muffins	Stuffed Acorn Squash	Fruit Salad with Mint and Lime Dressing	Sea Bass with Mediterranean Vegetables
19	Banana and Walnut Smoothie	Carrot and Ginger Soup	Sliced Apples with Almond Butter	Tofu Scramble with Vegetables
20	Greek Yogurt with Honey and Almonds	Broccoli and Potato Soup	Rice Paper Rolls with Avocado and Mango	Pork Chops with Peach Salsa
21	Sweet Potato and Kale Hash	Pumpkin Soup with Coconut Milk	Melon and Prosciutto Bites	Lemon Herb Roasted Chicken
22	Apple-Cinnamon Oat Porridge	Turkey and Vegetable Stew	Rice Paper Rolls with Avocado and Mango	Turkey Burger with Avocado
23	Sweet Potato and Chickpea Stew	Eggplant Parmesan Casserole	Sliced Apples with Almond Butter	Shrimp and Asparagus Stir Fry
24	Cottage Cheese with Pineapple Chunks	Pea and Ham Hock Soup	Tomato Bruschetta on Whole Grain Bread	Grilled Tilapia with Mango Salsa
25	Pumpkin Spice Oatmeal	Cauliflower Steak with Herb Sauce	Veggie Nori Rolls	Meatloaf with Turkey and Quinoa
26	Scrambled Tofu with Spinach and Tomatoes	Broccoli and Potato Soup	Tomato Bruschetta on Whole Grain Bread	Slow Cooker Pulled Pork
27	Pear and Ginger Overnight Oats	Sweet Potato and Chickpea Stew	Baked Kale Chips	Chicken Fajitas with Whole Wheat Tortillas
28	Apple-Cinnamon Oat Porridge	Spicy Black Bean Soup	Rice Paper Rolls with Avocado and Mango	Steamed Brown Rice

FREE GIFT

Thank you! Discover your gift inside! Dive into a rich assortment of DASH Diet for Beginners recipes for added inspiration. Gift it or share the PDF effortlessly with friends and family via a single click on WhatsApp or other social platforms. Bon appétit!

CONCLUSION OUTLINE

As we come to the end of our culinary journey with the "Pancreatitis Cookbook," it's time to reflect on the steps we've taken towards a lifestyle that supports the health of your pancreas. We've navigated through a collection of recipes designed to be gentle on your digestive system while still being full of flavor and nutrition.

Let's revisit the key takeaways. The dishes in this cookbook have been crafted to be low in fat, particularly avoiding the types of fats that are harder for a compromised pancreas to process. We've emphasized the importance of incorporating lean proteins, fibrous fruits and vegetables, and whole grains, which provide the essential nutrients your body needs without overburdening your pancreas.

We've discovered that a pancreatitis-friendly diet doesn't mean a bland or monotonous one. From the energizing breakfasts to the satisfying main courses, each recipe has been developed to delight your palate and support your health. Treats and snacks have also been carefully considered, because balance and enjoyment are key components of any sustainable diet.

This book is more than a collection of recipes; it's a guide to help you make conscious food choices every day. Following a pancreatitis diet means being mindful of the ingredients you use, reading nutritional labels with care, and being cognizant of portion sizes.

Remember, flexibility is at the heart of this diet. Feel free to substitute ingredients that may not suit you with those that do, keeping in mind the nutritional guidelines that support your condition. It's not just about avoiding certain foods; it's about embracing a variety of nutrient-dense foods that can aid in your healing and well-being.

Take your dietary changes one meal at a time. Start with a single recipe, master it, and then expand your menu. Gradually, you'll build a collection of go-to dishes that are both pancreas-friendly and delicious.

If you're ever uncertain or need to tailor recipes to your specific health needs, don't hesitate to consult with a dietitian or healthcare provider. They are your partners in health, ready to support you as you navigate your dietary needs.

In conclusion, this cookbook marks the beginning of a thoughtful way of eating that can enhance your quality of life. It's about celebrating food, enjoying the process of cooking, and finding comfort in the knowledge that you are nourishing your body in the best way possible. So, let's put on that apron and begin this adventure in healthy cooking. Your pancreas—and your taste buds—will be grateful.

REFERENCES

1. American Pancreatic Association. (2023). Nutrition Advice & Recipes. https://pancreasclub.com/patients/nutrition-advice-recipes/

2. Pancreatitis Supporters Network. (2023). Diet and Pancreatitis. https://pancreatitis.org.uk/diet-and-pancreatitis/

3. National Pancreas Foundation. (2023). Diet and Nutrition. https://pancreasfoundation.org/patient-information/diet-and-nutrition/

4. Gastroenterological Society of Australia. (2023). Pancreatic Disease. https://gastro.org.au/health-professionals/guidelines/pancreatic-disease/

5. Mayo Clinic. (2023). Pancreatitis Diet: What's a Low-Fat Recipe? https://www.mayoclinic.org/diseases-conditions/pancreatitis/expert-answers/faq-20058485

6. Pancreatic Cancer Action Network. (2023). Diet and Nutrition. https://pancan.org/facing-pancreatic-cancer/diet-and-nutrition/

7. Johns Hopkins Medicine. (2023). Pancreatitis Diet. https://www.hopkinsmedicine.org/health/conditions-and-diseases/pancreatitis/pancreatitis-diet

8. The Pancreatitis Diet Bible. Kerr, G. (2015). ISBN: 978-1500124625.

9. Dietitian's Guide to Chronic Pancreatitis. Wilson, L. (2021). ISBN: 978-1532182557.

10. Cleveland Clinic. (2023). Chronic Pancreatitis: Management and Treatment. https://my.clevelandclinic.org/health/diseases/15806-pancreatitis-management-and-treatment

APPENDIX 1:
MEASUREMENT CONVERSION CHART

U.S. SYSTEM	METRIC
1 inch	2.54 centimeters
1 fluid ounce	29.57 milliliters
1 pint (16 ounces)	473.18 milliliters, 2 cups
1 quart (32 ounces)	1 liter, 4 cups
1 gallon (128 ounces)	4 liters, 16 cups
1 pound (16 ounces)	437.5 grams (0.4536 kilogram), 473.18 milliliters
1 ounces	2 tablespoons, 28 grams
1 cup (8 ounces)	237 milliliters
1 teaspoon	5 milliliters
1 tablespoon	15 milliliters (3 teaspoons)
Fahrenheit (subtract 32 and divide by 1.8 to get Celsius)	Centigrade (multiply by 1.8 and add 32 to get Fahrenheit)

APPENDIX 2:
INDEX OF RECIPES

NOTES

NOTES

Made in the USA
Las Vegas, NV
13 September 2024

95213314R00052